Landmark Cases in Forensic Psychiatry

Landmark Cases in Forensic Psychiatry

Edited by

Elizabeth Ford, MD

Clinical Associate Professor of Psychiatry
Director, Forensic Psychiatry Fellowship
New York University School of Medicine
Director, Division of Forensic Psychiatry
Bellevue Hospital Center
New York, New York

Merrill Rotter, MD

Director, Division of Law and Psychiatry
Associate Clinical Professor of Psychiatry
Albert Einstein School of Medicine
Bronx, New York

UNIVERSITY PRESS

Oxford University Press is a department of the University of
Oxford. It furthers the University's objective of excellence in research,
scholarship, and education by publishing worldwide.

Oxford   New York
Auckland   Cape Town   Dar es Salaam   Hong Kong   Karachi
Kuala Lumpur   Madrid   Melbourne   Mexico City   Nairobi
New Delhi   Shanghai   Taipei   Toronto

With offices in
Argentina   Austria   Brazil   Chile   Czech Republic   France   Greece
Guatemala   Hungary   Italy   Japan   Poland   Portugal   Singapore
South Korea   Switzerland   Thailand   Turkey   Ukraine   Vietnam

Oxford is a registered trademark of Oxford University Press
in the UK and certain other countries.

Published in the United States of America by
Oxford University Press
198 Madison Avenue, New York, NY 10016

© Oxford University Press 2014

All rights reserved. No part of this publication may be reproduced, stored in
a retrieval system, or transmitted, in any form or by any means, without the prior
permission in writing of Oxford University Press, or as expressly permitted by law,
by license, or under terms agreed with the appropriate reproduction rights organization.
Inquiries concerning reproduction outside the scope of the above should be sent to the
Rights Department, Oxford University Press, at the address above.

You must not circulate this work in any other form
and you must impose this same condition on any acquirer.

Library of Congress Cataloging-in-Publication Data
Landmark cases in forensic psychiatry / edited by Elizabeth Ford, Merrill Rotter.
   p. ; cm.
Includes bibliographical references and index.
ISBN 978–0–19–934465–9 (alk. paper)
I. Ford, Elizabeth (Elizabeth B.), editor of compilation.   II. Rotter, Merrill, editor of compilation.
[DNLM: 1. Forensic Psychiatry—methods—Case Reports. W 740]
RA1148
614'.15—dc23
2014000080

This material is not intended to be, and should not be considered, a substitute for medical or other
professional advice. Treatment for the conditions described in this material is highly dependent on
the individual circumstances. And, while this material is designed to offer accurate information with
respect to the subject matter covered and to be current as of the time it was written, research and
knowledge about medical and health issues is constantly evolving and dose schedules for medications
are being revised continually, with new side effects recognized and accounted for regularly. Readers
must therefore always check the product information and clinical procedures with the most up-to-date
published product information and data sheets provided by the manufacturers and the most recent
codes of conduct and safety regulation. The publisher and the authors make no representations or
warranties to readers, express or implied, as to the accuracy or completeness of this material. Without
limiting the foregoing, the publisher and the authors make no representations or warranties as to the
accuracy or efficacy of the drug dosages mentioned in the material. The authors and the publisher do
not accept, and expressly disclaim, any responsibility for any liability, loss or risk that may be claimed
or incurred as a consequence of the use and/or application of any of the contents of this material.

CONTENTS

Alphabetical List of Cases   xi
Contributors   xv
Introduction   xix

SECTION I: Mental Health Practice Guidelines
Chapter 1: Confidentiality and Privilege   3
    In re Lifschutz   3
    Doe v. Roe   4
    Whalen v. Roe   5
    In re Subpoena Served upon Zuniga   5
    State v. Andring   6
    Commonwealth v. Kobrin   7
    Menendez v. Superior Court   8
    Jaffee v. Redmond   8
Chapter 2: Informed Consent   10
    Natanson v. Kline   10
    Canterbury v. Spence   11
    Kaimowitz v. Department of Mental Health for the State of Michigan   11
    Truman v. Thomas   12
    Clites v. Iowa   13
    Zinermon v. Burch   14
Chapter 3: Duty to Protect   15
    Tarasoff v. Regents   15
    Lipari v. Sears   16
    Petersen v. Washington   17
    Jablonski v. U.S.   17
    Naidu v. Laird   18
Chapter 4: Expert Testimony   20
    Frye v. U.S.   20
    State v. Hurd   21
    People v. Shirley   21

  Rock v. Arkansas 22
  Daubert v. Merrell Dow Pharmaceuticals 23
  General Electric v. Joiner 23
  Kumho Tire Co. v. Carmichael 24
Chapter 5: Questions on Mental Health Practice Guidelines 25

SECTION II: Institutional Treatment Guidelines

Chapter 6: Civil Commitment 43
  Lake v. Cameron 43
  Baxstrom v. Herold 44
  Lessard v. Schmidt 45
  O'Connor v. Donaldson 45
  Addington v. Texas 46
  Parham v. J.R. 47
Chapter 7: Right to Die 48
  Cruzan v. Director of Missouri Department of Mental Health 48
  Washington v. Glucksberg 49
  Vacco v. Quill 50
Chapter 8: Right to Treatment 51
  Rouse v. Cameron 51
  Wyatt v. Stickney 52
  Youngberg v. Romeo 52
Chapter 9: Right to Refuse Treatment 54
  Application of the President and Directors of Georgetown University 54
  Superintendent of Belchertown State School et al. v. Joseph Saikewicz 55
  In the Matter of the Guardianship of Richard Roe, III 55
  Rennie v. Klein 56
  Rogers v. Commissioner 57
Chapter 10: Questions on Institutional Treatment Guidelines 59

SECTION III: Child and Adolescent Issues

Chapter 11: Child Abuse Reporting 73
  Landeros v. Flood 73
  People v. Stritzinger 74
  DeShaney v. Winnebago 75
Chapter 12: Child Custody and Parental Competencies 76
  Painter v. Bannister 76
  Santosky v. Kramer 77
Chapter 13: Juvenile Rights 78
  In re Gault 78
  Graham v. Florida 79
  Miller v. Alabama 80

Chapter 14: EAHCA (Education for All Handicapped Children Act);
    IDEA (Individuals with Disabilities Education Act)   81
        Hendrick Hudson Board of Education v. Rowley   81
        Irving Independent School District v. Tatro   82
Chapter 15: Questions on Child and Adolescent Issues   84

SECTION IV: Tort Law
Chapter 16: ADA/Disability   97
    Carter v. General Motors   97
    Bragdon v. Abbott   98
    Pennsylvania v. Yeskey   99
    Olmstead v. Zimring   99
    Toyota v. Williams   100
    Hargrave v. Vermont   101
    U.S. v. Georgia   102
Chapter 17: Emotional Harm   103
    Dillon v. Legg   103
    Thing v. La Chusa   104
Chapter 18: Health Insurance   105
    Aetna v. McCabe   105
    Mazza v. Medical Mutual Insurance Company of North Carolina   106
    Wickline v. State   106
    Wilson v. Blue Cross of Southern California   107
    Corcoran v. United Healthcare, Inc.   108
    New York State Conference of Blue Cross and Blue Shield Plans et al. v. Travelers Insurance Co. et al.   109
    Dukes v. U.S. Healthcare, Inc.   109
    Aetna v. Davila   110
Chapter 19: Sexual Harassment   112
    Meritor Savings Bank v. Vinson   112
    Harris v. Forklift Systems, Inc.   113
    Oncale v. Sundowner Offshore Services, Inc.   114
Chapter 20: Sex   115
    Roy v. Hartogs   115
Chapter 21: Questions on Tort Law   116

SECTION V: Criminal Law and Incarceration
Chapter 22: Criminal Procedure   131
    Miranda v. Arizona   131
    North Carolina v. Alford   132
    Colorado v. Connelly   132
    Robinson v. California   133
    Powell v. Texas   134

Chapter 23: Criminal Competencies   135
    Dusky v. U.S.   135
    Wilson v. U.S.   136
    Jackson v. Indiana   136
    Drope v. Missouri   137
    Godinez v. Moran   138
    Cooper v. Oklahoma   139
    Indiana v. Edwards   140

Chapter 24: Diminished Capacity   141
    People v. Patterson   141
    Ibn-Tamas v. U.S.   142
    People v. Saille   142
    Montana v. Egelhoff   143

Chapter 25: Insanity   144
    M'Naghten's Case   144
    Durham v. U.S.   145
    Washington v. U.S.   145
    Frendak v. U.S.   146
    Jones v. U.S.   147
    U.S. v. Torniero   147
    Foucha v. Louisiana   148
    Clark v. Arizona   149

Chapter 26: Prisoners' Rights   151
    Estelle v. Gamble   151
    Vitek v. Jones   152
    Washington v. Harper   152
    Riggins v. Nevada   153
    Farmer v. Brennan   154
    Sell v. U.S.   155
    Brown v. Plata   156

Chapter 27: Death Penalty   157
    Estelle v. Smith   157
    Ake v. Oklahoma   158
    Ford v. Wainwright   158
    Payne v. Tennessee   159
    State v. Perry   160
    Atkins v. Virginia   160
    Roper v. Simmons   161
    Panetti v. Quarterman   162

Chapter 28: Sex Offenders   163
    Specht v. Patterson   163
    Allen v. Illinois   164
    In re Young and Cunningham   164
    Kansas v. Hendricks   165
    McKune v. Lile   166
    Kansas v. Crane   167
    U.S. v. Comstock   168
Chapter 29: Questions on Criminal Law and Incarceration   169

Appendix A: The Bill of Rights and Fourteenth Amendment,
    U.S. Constitution   195
Appendix B: General Path to the U.S. Supreme Court   201
Appendix C: Geographic Boundaries of the U.S. and
    DC Circuit Courts of Appeal   203

Index   205

ALPHABETICAL LIST OF CASES

1. *Addington v. Texas*   46
2. *Aetna v. Davila*   110
3. *Aetna v. McCabe*   105
4. *Ake v. Oklahoma*   158
5. *Allen v. Illinois*   164
6. *Application of the President and Directors of Georgetown University*   54
7. *Atkins v. Virginia*   160
8. *Baxstrom v. Herold*   44
9. *Bragdon v. Abbott*   98
10. *Brown v. Plata*   156
11. *Canterbury v. Spence*   11
12. *Carter v. General Motors*   97
13. *Clark v. Arizona*   149
14. *Clites v. Iowa*   13
15. *Colorado v. Connelly*   132
16. *Commonwealth v. Kobrin*   7
17. *Cooper v. Oklahoma*   139
18. *Corcoran v. United Healthcare, Inc.*   108
19. *Cruzan v. Director of Missouri Department of Mental Health*   48
20. *Daubert v. Merrell Dow Pharmaceuticals*   23
21. *DeShaney v. Winnebago*   75
22. *Dillon v. Legg*   103
23. *Doe v. Roe*   4
24. *Drope v. Missouri*   137
25. *Dukes v. U.S. Healthcare, Inc.*   109
26. *Durham v. U.S.*   145
27. *Dusky v. U.S.*   135
28. *Estelle v. Gamble*   151
29. *Estelle v. Smith*   157
30. *Farmer v. Brennan*   154

31. *Ford v. Wainwright* 158
32. *Foucha v. Louisiana* 148
33. *Frendak v. U.S.* 146
34. *Frye v. U.S.* 20
35. *General Electric v. Joiner* 23
36. *Godinez v. Moran* 138
37. *Graham v. Florida* 79
38. *Hargrave v. Vermont* 101
39. *Harris v. Forklift Systems, Inc.* 113
40. *Hendrick Hudson Board of Education v. Rowley* 81
41. *Ibn-Tamas v. U.S.* 142
42. *In re Gault* 78
43. *In re Lifschutz* 3
44. *In the Matter of the Guardianship of Richard Roe, III* 55
45. *In re Young and Cunningham* 164
46. *In re Subpoena Served upon Zuniga* 5
47. *Indiana v. Edwards* 140
48. *Irving Independent School District v. Tatro* 82
49. *Jablonski v. U.S.* 17
50. *Jackson v. Indiana* 136
51. *Jaffee v. Redmond* 8
52. *Jones v. U.S.* 147
53. *Kaimowitz v. Department of Mental Health for the State of Michigan* 11
54. *Kansas v. Crane* 167
55. *Kansas v. Hendricks* 165
56. *Kumho Tire Co. v. Carmichael* 24
57. *Lessard v. Schmidt* 45
58. *Lake v. Cameron* 43
59. *Landeros v. Flood* 73
60. *Lipari v. Sears* 16
61. *Mazza v. Medical Mutual Insurance Company of North Carolina* 106
62. *McKune v. Lile* 166
63. *Menendez v. Superior Court* 8
64. *Meritor Savings Bank v. Vinson* 112
65. *Miller v. Alabama* 80
66. *Miranda v. Arizona* 131
67. *M'Naghten's Case* 144
68. *Montana v. Egelhoff* 143
69. *Natanson v. Kline* 10
70. *New York State Conference of Blue Cross and Blue Shield Plans et al. v. Travelers Insurance Co. et al.* 109

71. *North Carolina v. Alford*   132
72. *O'Connor v. Donaldson*   45
73. *Olmstead v. Zimring*   199
74. *Oncale v. Sundowner Offshore Services, Inc.*   114
75. *Painter v. Bannister*   76
76. *Panetti v. Quarterman*   162
77. *Parham v. J.R.*   47
78. *Payne v. Tennessee*   159
79. *Pennsylvania v. Yeskey*   99
80. *People v. Patterson*   141
81. *People v. Saille*   142
82. *People v. Shirley*   21
83. *People v. Stritzinger*   74
84. *Petersen v. Washington*   17
85. *Powell v. Texas*   134
86. *Rennie v. Klein*   56
87. *Riggins v. Nevada*   153
88. *Robinson v. California*   133
89. *Rock v. Arkansas*   22
90. *Rogers v. Commissioner*   57
91. *Roper v. Simmons*   161
92. *Rouse v. Cameron*   51
93. *Roy v. Hartogs*   115
94. *Santosky v. Kramer*   77
95. *Sell v. U.S.*   155
96. *Specht v. Patterson*   163
97. *State v. Andring*   6
98. *State v. Hurd*   21
99. *State v. Perry*   160
100. *Superintendent of Belchertown State School et al. v. Joseph Saikewicz*   55
101. *Tarasoff v. Regents*   15
101. *Thing v. La Chusa*   104
103. *Toyota v. Williams*   100
104. *Truman v. Thomas*   12
105. *U.S. v. Comstock*   168
106. *U.S. v. Georgia*   102
107. *U.S. v. Torniero*   147
108. *Vacco v. Quill*   50
109. *Vitek v. Jones*   152
110. *Washington v. Glucksberg*   49

111. *Washington v. Harper*   152
112. *Washington v. U.S.*   145
113. *Whalen v. Roe*   5
114. *Wickline v. State*   106
115. *Wilson v. Blue Cross of Southern California*   107
116. *Wilson v. U.S.*   136
117. *Wyatt v. Stickney*   52
118. *Youngberg v. Romeo*   52
119. *Zinermon v. Burch*   14

CONTRIBUTORS

Eraka Bath, MD
Director, Child Forensic Services
Assistant Professor, Department of Psychiatry
UCLA Neuropsychiatric Institute
[Chapters 1, 11]

Gregory Davis, MD
Attending Psychiatrist
Bellevue Hospital Center
Clinical Instructor in Psychiatry
New York University School of Medicine
[Chapter 2]

Elizabeth Ford, MD
Director, Division of Forensic Psychiatry
Bellevue Hospital Center
Training Director, Forensic Psychiatry Fellowship
Clinical Associate Professor of Psychiatry
New York University School of Medicine
[Chapters 6, 7, 13, 18]

Howard Forman, MD
Attending Physician
Division of Psychosomatic Medicine
Montefiore Medical Center
[Chapter 16]

Katya Frischer, MD
Associate Residency Director
Department of Psychiatry
Bronx Lebanon Hospital Center
Assistant Professor of Psychiatry

Albert Einstein College of Medicine of Yeshiva University
[Chapter 25]

Michael Greenspan, MD
Unit Chief
Zucker Hillside Hospital
North Shore–Long Island Jewish Health System
[Chapters 22, 24]

Matthew W. Grover, MD
Forensic Coordinator, Bronx Psychiatric Center
Assistant Site Supervisor, Forensic Psychiatry Fellowship
Albert Einstein College of Medicine of Yeshiva University
[Chapter 23]

Omar Khan, MD
Attending Psychiatrist
Bellevue Hospital Center
Clinical Instructor in Psychiatry
New York University School of Medicine
[Chapter 26]

S. Shane Konrad, MD
Clinical Assistant Professor of Psychiatry
New York University School of Medicine
[Chapter 1]

Andrew M. Kopelman, MD
Attending Psychiatrist
Bellevue Hospital Center
Clinical Instructor in Psychiatry
New York University School of Medicine
[Chapter 3]

Li-Wen G. Lee, MD
Clinical Assistant Professor of Psychiatry
Columbia University College of Physicians and Surgeons
[Chapter 28]

Andrew P. Levin, MD
Medical Director, Westchester Jewish Community Services
Assistant Clinical Professor of Psychiatry
Columbia University College of Physicians and Surgeons
[Chapter 19]

Rebecca Lewis, MD
Attending Psychiatrist
Bellevue Hospital Center Comprehensive Psychiatric Emergency Program
Clinical Instructor in Psychiatry
New York University School of Medicine
[Chapters 9, 26]

Amar Mehta, MD
Forensic Psychiatrist
San Quentin State Prison
[Chapters 17, 22]

Merrill Rotter, MD
Director, Forensic Services
Bronx Psychiatric Center
Medical Director, EAC-TASC Diversion Programs
Associate Clinical Professor of Psychiatry
Albert Einstein College of Medicine
[Chapters 18, 19, 20, 22]

Eileen P. Ryan, DO
Associate Professor of Psychiatry and Neurobehavioral Sciences
University of Virginia School of Medicine
[Chapters 12, 13]

Bryan C. Shelby, MD, JD
Attending Psychiatrist, Substance Abuse Treatment Program
Newington Veterans Hospital
Assistant Professor of Psychiatry
University of Connecticut Health Center School of Medicine
[Chapters 4, 18]

Shawn S. Sidhu, MD
Inpatient Attending Psychiatrist, Children's Psychiatric Center
Assistant Professor, University of New Mexico Department of Psychiatry
[Chapters 11, 14]

Scott Soloway, MD
Director, Manhattan/Correctional Assisted Outpatient Treatment Program
New York City Department of Health and Mental Hygiene
Clinical Assistant Professor of Psychiatry
New York University School of Medicine
[Chapter 4]

Tara Straka, MD
Attending Psychiatrist, Kirby Forensic Psychiatric Center
Clinical Instructor in Psychiatry
New York University School of Medicine
[Chapter 27]

Bipin Subedi, MD
Assistant Program Director, Forensic Psychiatry Fellowship
Clinical Instructor in Psychiatry
New York University School of Medicine
[Chapters 8, 26]

INTRODUCTION

ELIZABETH FORD AND MERRILL ROTTER

Forensic psychiatry (the interface of psychiatry and the law), forensic psychology, and mental health law are growing and evolving subspecialties in their respective larger disciplines. The fields are deeply rooted in the written opinions and holdings about mental health from various U.S. courts (with one exception—*M'Naghten's Case* of 1843), most important, the U.S. Supreme Court. These decisions cover topics as broad-reaching as informed consent and as narrow as sentencing guidelines for adolescents convicted of nonhomicide cases. The opinions are frequently lengthy and dense, with much revealed in the writing not only about the specific reasoning behind a decision but also about the sociopolitical climate at the time of the case and the political preferences of the appointed justices on the bench. The opinions can read easily like novels or more laboriously like legal textbooks. Regardless of the style or length, however, the substance of the decision is critical for some facet of the mental health system in this country. Without knowledge of the historical and legal precedents set by these cases, mental health practitioners are at a significant disadvantage.

Recognizing the importance of these holdings, the American Academy of Psychiatry and the Law (AAPL), the premier national organization in the United States for forensic psychiatrists, compiled a list of more than 100 cases representing the core of the specialty. Because the list was created more than 25 years ago, it has changed as new cases have been decided and others have become obsolete or outdated. However, the majority of the decisions remain essential to understanding why practitioners in mental health are legally required to practice as they do. Most, if not all, of the 43 American and 6 Canadian forensic psychiatry fellowship training programs, competitive subspecialty training programs available after completion of a

4-year psychiatry residency, incorporate discussion and study of the landmark cases into their yearlong didactics.

The American Board of Forensic Psychiatry was founded in 1976 to establish standards for competence in psychiatry and the law. The board administered its own examination and certified 253 diplomates until the American Board of Medical Specialties officially recognized the field of forensic psychiatry in 1992.[1] Since then, the American Board of Psychiatry and Neurology (ABPN) has been certifying specialists in the field of forensic psychiatry (the ABPN administered its first exam in 1994) and continues to sponsor a biannual written certification exam. Passing this increasingly rigorous exam following completion of a forensic psychiatry fellowship is considered evidence of one's competence and professionalism in the field and, much like general board certification in other areas of medicine, is a highly coveted accomplishment. Recertification is required every 10 years to maintain standing with the ABPN. The American Board of Forensic Psychology also administers a certification exam for forensic psychologists and has done so since 1947. Unlike the ABPN, this certification also involves work review and an oral examination.[2]

The emphasis that the ABPN certification and recertification exams have placed on knowledge of the landmark cases has evolved over the years. While various exams have encouraged or discouraged rote memorization of case names and jurisdictions, the impact of the holdings and accompanying reasoning on the practice of forensic psychiatry has always remained critical. In January 2013, the ABPN published a Content Outline for its 200-question, multiple-choice certification examination and highlighted the key areas of knowledge required. Included in that outline are 100 landmark cases covering the legal regulation of psychiatry, civil and criminal issues, the death penalty, corrections and correctional health care, basic law, children and family issues, and special issues in forensic psychiatry.[3]

Sources of study for landmark cases have typically taken the form of a compilation of summaries and/or discussion of cases in forensic psychiatry textbooks,[4,5] in mental health law texts,[6,7] and in the course materials for the annual 3-day American Academy of Psychiatry and the Law Forensic Psychiatry Review Course.[8] A set of landmark case "flash cards" was available for a brief period (2005–2010) that had been created by the New York University Forensic Psychiatry Fellowship Class of 2005.[9] The majority of the texts of the opinions themselves are easily accessible online. While this collection of sources is and will continue to be extremely useful, and was invaluable in the preparation of this book, it does not uniquely focus on the landmark cases (with the exception of the defunct flash cards and the lengthy court opinions) in a way that is clearly aimed at both developing a greater understanding of their impact and preparing for an examination. This book was written to fill that gap.

We have designed this book with forensic psychiatry and psychology trainees and practicing clinicians in mind. There are five sections that define broad topic areas, included in which are multiple chapters with more narrow areas of focus. We classified cases based on our interpretation of the most important holding for each case. While this classification system tends to align with the way other sources have grouped cases, there are some changes that we think will help the reader better contextualize the narrative and practical implications of the cases.

All the cases listed in the 2013 ABPN Content Outline are included, as are other cases that we find particularly important for understanding a topic. Not all the cases will seem relevant, and indeed some have been overturned by higher rulings, but when preparing for a board exam, we find it better to be more inclusive rather than less.

We have tried to create summaries that are easy to follow and get quickly to the point. They are presented chronologically in each chapter so that the reader can understand the evolution of ideas on a particular topic. We have also turned the main holding of each case into a "yes or no" question to allow readers to get even more quickly to the point. Bear in mind that in order to provide concise summaries for study purposes, many of the details of each individual case have been excluded. For those who would like to review the cases in more detail, we have provided a free online link to the full text of each case.

Although this study guide is not designed in any way to be a primer on law or the legal system, the cases discussed have all been adjudicated within the context of state or federal court systems, most frequently the US Supreme Court. This body is the highest federal court in the United States and has as a major task deciding cases for which it grants certiorari (a willingness to hear a case) based on an interpretation of the U.S. Constitution. The Bill of Rights (the first ten amendments to the Constitution, ratified in 1791) and the Fourteenth Amendment form the basis for Court's decisions involving psychiatry and are listed in Appendix A. Appendix B presents a very general framework about state and federal court systems in the United States. It is not necessary to know the exact path a case took to get to the Supreme Court, but the various arguments presented along the way for and against a particular outcome are important. It is also useful to know to which jurisdiction a case applies (e.g., only a particular state district, all of the states represented in a court of appeals circuit).

The addition of a robust assembly of multiple-choice questions at the end of each section will help test the reader's knowledge and test-taking skills;

we hope the detailed explanations of each answer will also help cement that knowledge in a lasting way. The questions are designed to mimic ABPN-style questions (e.g., no "except" questions, no "A and B, A and C" answers) but should be used only for guidance and practice. The questions are not drawn from actual board exams but have been created by the editors and contributors to be as clear and as helpful as possible.

We are grateful to the leaders in forensic psychiatry who have helped to shape this field into a well-respected and highly rigorous discipline that is deserving of the ABPN's certification. A special thank you to the other members of the NYU Fellowship Class of 2005 (Drs. Scott Soloway, Eraka Bath, and Manuel Lopez-Leon) and Dr. Henry Weinstein for all of the hard upfront work on Flash Forensics and their continued support since then. Finally, we are extremely grateful to the many forensic psychiatry fellows who have passed through our respective fellowship programs and who have inspired and taught us to be better teachers. Thank you all for your help with this project.

REFERENCES

1 Prentice SE. A history of subspecialization in forensic psychiatry. *Bull Am Acad Psychiatry Law* 1995; 23(2): 195–203.
2 American Board of Forensic Psychology. http://www.abfp.com/brochure.asp. Accessed November 6, 2013.
3 ABPN. Subspecialty Certification Examination in Forensic Psychiatry, 2013 Content Blueprint. www.abpn.com/downloads/content_outlines/Initial Cert/2 013-FP-blueprint-010413-EE-MR.pdf. Issued January 4, 2013.
4 Rosner R, ed. *Principles and practice of forensic psychiatry*. 2nd ed. London: Arnold. 2003.
5 Simon RI, Gold L. *Textbook of forensic psychiatry*. 2nd ed. Arlington, VA: American Psychiatric Publishing, 2010.
6 Perlin MI. *Mental disability law: Cases and materials*. 2nd ed. Durham, NC: Carolina Academic Press, 2005
7 Slobogin C, Rai A. *Law and the mental health system: Civil and criminal aspects*. 5th ed. St. Paul, MN: West Academic Publishing. 2008.
8 Resnick P. *Annual forensic psychiatry review course*. Bloomfield, CT: American Academy of Psychiatry and the Law, 2012
9 Ford E, Bath E, Lopez-Leon M, Soloway S. *Flash ForensicsTM: U.S. landmark cases about psychiatry and the law*. 2nd ed. New York, NY. 2008.

SECTION I

Mental Health Practice Guidelines

The cases included in this section address topics related to the general practice of medicine and psychiatry. Issues such as informed consent and mandated reporting to protect vulnerable individuals are now nearly universal concepts for practicing physicians. Psychiatrists, as practitioners of a medical specialty that is legally regulated, should be familiar with their state statutory requirements and understand the reasoning behind the decisions. For example, confidentiality and its legal corollary, privilege, are both critical elements of providing mental health care, yet they were not clearly recognized as such by the law until 35 years ago. Informed consent, now a guiding principle in almost every doctor–patient interaction, is also a relatively new phenomenon.

Chapters 3 and 4 in this section ("Duty to Protect" and "Expert Testimony") also relate to topics that extend outside of the mental health professions. Child abuse reporting, for example, is not specific to psychiatry. Expert testimony, recognized by the American Medical Association (AMA) as the practice of medicine, is not specific to psychiatry. But psychiatrists, as well as mental health clinicians in other professional disciplines such as psychology and social work, may find themselves in mandated reporting situations or expert witness situations that directly relate to the holdings in the cases described in this section.

CHAPTER 1

Confidentiality and Privilege

S. SHANE KONRAD AND ERAKA BATH

IN RE LIFSCHUTZ, 487 P.2D 557 (1970)

Link to case: http://www.stanford.edu/group/psylawseminar/Lifschutz.htm

Question: Can a psychiatrist assert privilege for information gathered in the course of treatment, when the patient has waived privilege?

Answer: No.

Joseph Housek was in treatment with his psychiatrist, Dr. Joseph Lifschutz, 10 years prior to filing a civil lawsuit in a California court for an alleged assault by a high school student. Mr. Housek claimed mental and emotional distress. The student defendant's attorney found out about this prior treatment and subpoenaed Dr. Lifschutz and his records. Dr. Lifschutz appeared in court as a witness but refused to provide medical records or give testimony about Mr. Housek's treatment. Dr. Lifschutz claimed that the court order was invalid as unconstitutionally infringing on his personal right of privacy, his right to effectively practice his profession, and the constitutional privacy rights of his patients. Dr. Lifschutz was found in contempt and jailed for several days based on the reasoning that Mr. Housek had waived his privacy privilege by initiating the lawsuit and asking for damages for pain and suffering, making his emotional state an issue. Dr. Lifschutz filed for habeas corpus. The California Supreme Court confirmed the contempt of court finding, and the writ of habeas corpus was denied. The court found that the need for confidentiality in psychotherapy must be balanced with society's need for determining the truth. It stated that the patient, not the therapist, had the right to privacy, and therefore the exclusive ability to waive that right.

DOE V. ROE, 93. MISC. 2D 201 (1977)

Link to case: http://scholar.google.com/scholar_case?case=4446229919103114898

Question: Is patient confidentiality violated by the publication of information, without informed consent, obtained during psychiatric treatment?

Answer: Yes.

Jane Doe (a pseudonym) sued her former psychiatrist, Dr. Jane Roe (also a pseudonym), and Dr. Roe's psychologist husband for damages, alleging that they unlawfully violated her privacy by publishing a book that included information obtained during Ms. Doe's couples psychotherapy sessions. The book was released years after the treatment and included "verbatim and extensively the patient's thoughts, feelings, emotions, fantasies, and biographies." Ms. Doe requested to have the publication stopped. The trial court, without a jury, held that the publication should be stopped and Ms. Doe was awarded $20,000 in compensatory damages. The New York State Supreme Court found that licensing regulations and professional ethical codes required that information shared in the physician–patient relationship be kept confidential. The court noted that "patients could only reveal their most intimate and socially unacceptable instincts and urges, immature wishes, and perverse sexual thoughts in an atmosphere of unusual trust."

The court rejected Dr. Roe's rebuttals that she had obtained oral consent from Ms. Doe, that the book contributed to scientific knowledge, and that she had adequately disguised Ms. Doe's identity. The court also found that privacy rights of patients limited free speech rights. The court rejected punitive damages because Dr. Roe's actions were not willful, malicious, or wanton as required by law but "merely stupid." Of note, Dr. Roe's husband was held equally liable. Even though he was not Ms. Doe's psychiatrist, he helped to get the book written, advertised, and distributed and was therefore a "willing violator of the patient's rights."

WHALEN V. ROE, 429 U.S. 589 (1977)

Link to case: http://caselaw.lp.findlaw.com/scripts/getcase.pl?navby=case&court=us&vol=429&page=589

Question: Can a state constitutionally collect personal information about patients who are receiving prescriptions for narcotics?

Answer: Yes.

In 1972, the New York state legislature enacted the New York State Controlled Substances Act because of concern that certain prescription drugs were being unlawfully diverted. The act required doctors to fill out forms for Schedule II prescription drugs. The prescribing doctor kept one copy, one copy was sent to the pharmacy, and a third copy was sent to the state department of health. The forms included personal information such as the patient's name, age, and address. Physicians and patients brought an action challenging the constitutionality of this statute. Even though the statute prohibited public disclosure of the patient's identity, the plaintiffs voiced concern about the privacy of patients who had their personal information stored in a centralized computer. The district court found the New York law unconstitutional, stating that some patients may decline necessary medications out of concern that misuse of the computerized data could cause them to be stigmatized as "drug addicts." An appeal was taken up by the U.S. Supreme Court, which reversed the district court decision. The Court held that the requirements of the act did not violate a "constitutionally protected 'zone of privacy.'" The Court found that the statute evidenced "a proper concern with, and protection of, the individual's interest in privacy" and that the "remote possibility" of potential abuses of data accumulation and disclosure was not sufficient to establish an invasion of any rights or liberties protected by the Fourteenth Amendment.

IN RE SUBPOENA SERVED UPON ZUNIGA, 714 F.2D 632 (1983)

Link to case: http://www.leagle.com/decision/19831346714F2d632_11238

Question: Can a psychotherapist's refusal to respond to a grand jury subpoena lead to a ruling of contempt?

Answer: Yes.

In a case investigating insurance fraud, the grand jury for the Eastern District of Michigan issued a subpoena commanding a psychiatrist, Dr. Jorge Zuniga, to appear before the grand jury and produce the following records: (1) redacted copies of patient files indicating patient name, date of service, type of psychotherapy session rendered (i.e., full, half, brief), and amount billed; (2) original ledger cards for patients; and (3) originals of any intraoffice forms in support of services rendered and date thereof. Dr. Zuniga refused to produce these records and filed a motion in the district court to quash the subpoena. He was found in civil contempt and ordered into custody of the U.S. Marshal Service pending the outcome of the appeal. The U.S. Court of Appeals for the Sixth Circuit affirmed and held that the information Dr. Zuniga was required to release to the court was not protected by psychotherapist-patient privilege. The appellate court also found that release of this information to the grand jury was not a violation of patients' privacy rights given the "veil of secrecy" in grand jury proceedings. The court also found that Dr. Zuniga could not invoke his Fifth Amendment privilege against self-incrimination to defend his refusal to release records because he was incorporated and not functioning as a private individual in this situation.

STATE V. ANDRING, 342 N.W.2D 128 (1984)

Link to case: http://scholar.google.com/scholar_case?case=18146708613969658932

Question: Does the scope of the physician–patient privilege extend to group therapy?

Answer: Yes.

David Andring had been criminally charged in Minnesota for sexual misconduct with his 10-year-old stepdaughter and 11-year-old niece. While awaiting trial, he voluntarily entered a treatment facility where he received individual and group therapy for alcohol treatment. He openly disclosed the sexual abuse in both individual and group therapy settings. When prosecutors became aware of his treatment, they moved to disclose his treatment records. While the trial court denied the admittance of his intake and individual therapy records, it did permit release of his group therapy records. Mr. Andring appealed and argued that the Federal Comprehensive Alcohol Abuse and Alcoholism Prevention, Treatment and Rehabilitation Act Amendments of 1974 ("federal alcohol treatment act") preempted the state's mandated reporting of abuse. The Supreme Court of Minnesota reversed the decision, finding that physician–patient privilege *did* extend to group therapy sessions, especially because the abuse was already known and his group therapy session records were not necessary to proceed with the criminal prosecution. The court noted that violation of physician–patient privilege from the group therapy sessions would not serve to further protect the children. The court also ruled that the federal alcohol treatment act, which extends a broad privilege to protect a patient's identity, diagnosis, prognosis, and treatment, does not trump the state-mandated reporting of child abuse.

COMMONWEALTH V. KOBRIN, 479 N.E.2D 674 (1985)

Link to case: http://scholar.google.com/scholar_case?case=18127391409676670050

Question: Can a limited set of records be subpoenaed from a psychiatrist to investigate billing fraud?

Answer: Yes.

A grand jury in Massachusetts subpoenaed complete records of patients whose cases were being investigated for alleged fraud violations of the Medicaid False Claim Act. In this particular case, 27 patients of a psychiatrist named Dr. Kennard Kobrin objected to the disclosure of their personal medical records, citing invasion of privacy. Dr. Kobrin refused to provide the records, but a superior court judge ordered the records to be produced. Dr. Kobrin then produced "sanitized" copies of the patients' charts, citing his patients' rights to exercise their psychotherapist-patient privilege. He was held in contempt, and his records were seized. The Supreme Court of Massachusetts found that both the government's need to know and the patients' confidentiality could be accommodated. The court held that Kobrin could submit records documenting "times and lengths of patient appointments, fees, patient diagnoses, treatment plans and recommendations, and somatic therapies." This limited information would allow for a legitimate investigation. Those portions of records reflecting any patient's thoughts, feelings, impressions, or containing the substance of any psychotherapeutic dialogue, or exposing personal relationships were of no concern to legitimate investigation.

MENENDEZ V. SUPERIOR COURT, 834 P.2D. 786 (1992)

Link to case: http://scholar.google.com/scholar_case?case=11801048403762594860

Question: Does the psychotherapist-patient privilege apply to treatment records regarding dangerousness?

Answer: No.

In this highly publicized case, brothers Erik and Lyle Menendez were charged with murdering their parents. A magistrate in the Municipal Court of the Beverly Hills Judicial District of Los Angeles County issued a search warrant authorizing a search of the office and residence of Leon Jerome Oziel, PhD (a clinical psychologist who was Erik and Lyle's psychotherapist) and seizure of specified items if found therein, including audiotape recordings containing information relating to the killings. The brothers filed a petition in support of Dr. Oziel, who claimed that audiotapes he made of his notes and of sessions with the Menendez brothers were covered by psychotherapist-patient privilege. On several tapes there was documentation of the brothers' threats of harm to Dr. Oziel, and on others there were threats to his lover and his wife. A California superior court and then the California Supreme Court found that some of the audiotapes could be disclosed. The California Supreme Court found that the tapes met the "dangerous person" exception to the therapist-patient privilege and that information is privileged unless it contains information indicating a patient is dangerous and unless disclosure of dangerousness is necessary to prevent harm. The "dangerous person" exception requires that the psychotherapist have reasonable cause for belief of dangerousness. It does not demand that the patient must be dangerous to a person other than the psychotherapist—although in this case the patients were.

JAFFEE V. REDMOND, 518 U.S. 1 (1996)

Link to case: http://caselaw.lp.findlaw.com/scripts/getcase.pl?navby=case&court=us&vol=518&page=1

Question: Should federal courts identify a psychotherapist-patient privilege?

Answer: Yes.

Mary Lu Redmond was the first police officer to respond to a "fight in progress" call at an apartment complex. According to Redmond, Ricky

Allen was brandishing a knife when he came out of the apartment and disregarded her repeated commands to drop the weapon. Redmond shot and killed Allen when she believed he was about to stab the man he was chasing. Carrie Jaffee was the special administrator of Allen's estate and filed suit in federal district court alleging that Redmond had violated Allen's constitutional rights by using excessive force. After this traumatic event, Redmond participated in about 50 counseling sessions with Karen Beyer, a licensed clinical social worker. Beyer and Redmond refused requests to share information discussed in their sessions with the court. They asserted that this information was protected against involuntary disclosure by a psychotherapist-patient privilege. The district judge rejected this argument and advised the jury that Beyer's refusal to turn over her notes had no "legal justification," and the jury could presume that the records were unfavorable to Redmond. The U.S. Court of Appeals for the Seventh Circuit reversed and remanded for a new trial. The court concluded that "reason and experience," the touchstones for acceptance of a privilege under Rule 501 of the Federal Rules of Evidence, compelled recognition of a psychotherapist-patient privilege. "Reason tells us that psychotherapists and patients share a unique relationship, in which the ability to communicate freely without the fear of public disclosure is the key to successful treatment." As to experience, the court observed that all 50 states have adopted some form of the psychotherapist-patient privilege. The U.S. Supreme Court affirmed the appellate court ruling.

CHAPTER 2

Informed Consent

GREGORY DAVIS

NATANSON V. KLINE, 350 P.2D 1093 (1960)

Link to case: http://scholar.google.com/scholar_case?case=1590825446079418783

Question: Is informed consent required for nonnegligent physician care?

Answer: Yes.

Irma Natanson sustained burns from cobalt radiation therapy as part of her treatment for breast cancer. She filed a malpractice suit against her radiologist, Dr. Kline, claiming that she was not adequately informed of the risks of treatment beforehand. Although the trial court found that the doctor was not negligent, upon appeal the Kansas Supreme Court found that the trial court committed error in not providing to the jury specific instructions defining the amount of disclosure sufficient for a physician to obtain informed consent. According to the appellate court, elements required for informed consent include the nature of the illness, the proposed treatment, alternative treatment, the probability of success, and the risks involved. Ms. Natanson requested instruction to the jury that a physician had a duty to make a full disclosure to the patient of all matters within his knowledge affecting the interests of the patient. The Kansas Supreme Court found that the requested instruction was too broad, stating that a physician's duty is limited to disclosures that a "reasonable medical practitioner" would make under similar circumstances. This standard assumes that a consensus exists within the medical community and allows the physician to use his or her medical judgment.

CANTERBURY V. SPENCE, 464 F.2D 772 (1972)

Link to case: http://scholar.google.com/scholar_case?case=16106013819601769055

Question: Can a physician be liable for malpractice if he or she fails to disclose severe, although rare, risks inherent in a medical procedure?

Answer: Yes.

Jerry Canterbury underwent a laminectomy performed by Dr. Spence as part of an evaluation of his back pain. The day after the surgery, Mr. Canterbury fell from his unattended hospital bed, leading to paraplegia and incontinence. He filed suit for negligence, alleging in part that he was not informed of the 1% risk of paralysis that Dr. Spence testified would be anticipated with a laminectomy. Dr. Spence said that communication of risk of paralysis was not good medical practice because it might deter patients from undergoing needed surgery. After an initial finding for Dr. Spence, the case was brought before the DC Court of Appeals, which reversed and elaborated on the scope of the disclosure requirement necessary for informed consent. The court reasoned that a professional medical standard such as described in *Natanson v. Kline* is at odds with a patient's prerogative to decide on a projected treatment. In its view, the patient's right to self-decision shapes the boundaries of disclosure. Based on medical training and experience, the court said, a physician can sense how much an average, reasonable patient would want to know. The court defined the standard for disclosure as being based on what a "reasonable person" would find material to decision making, including serious, but rare, risks. It noted two exceptions as an incapacitated person in an emergency situation and if disclosure itself may do harm.

KAIMOWITZ V. DEPARTMENT OF MENTAL HEALTH FOR THE STATE OF MICHIGAN, NO. 73-19434-AW, MICH. CIR. CT., WAYNE CO. (1973)

Link to case: http://psychrights.org/Research/Legal/InformedConsent/KaimowitzvMichDeptMH%28MichCir1973%29.pdf

Question: Does involuntary commitment to a state psychiatric facility preclude providing adequate informed consent for experimental psychosurgery?

Answer: Yes.

John Doe had been committed to the Ionia State hospital in 1955 under a criminal sexual psychopathy law in Michigan. Mr. Doe provided informed consent to participate in an approved study of uncontrolled aggression. The study utilized experimental techniques and compared amygdaloid surgery to administration of the drug cyproterone. A third party, Mr. Kaimowitz, filed a writ of habeas corpus alleging that Mr. Doe was being illegally detained for surgery. The court directed Mr. Doe's release but also opined about the legality of the consent process. The court reasoned that when compared with accepted treatments, experimental psychosurgery could have substantial risk with no known benefits. It noted that informed consent should be closely scrutinized for procedures with a high risk-to-benefit ratio and should be competent, knowing, and voluntary. The court referenced the Nuremberg Code statement that experimental subjects should be able to exercise free power of choice without force, deceit, duress, or coercion. The court concluded that involuntarily confined patients, such as Mr. Doe in a state hospital, live in an "inherently coercive" situation that makes it impossible to give voluntary consent for a risky procedure. Of note, the ruling applied only to experimental psychosurgery; the court held that an involuntarily detained mental patient could possibly give adequate consent for accepted medical procedures.

TRUMAN V. THOMAS, 611 P.2D 902 (1980)

Link to case: http://scholar.google.com/scholar_case?case=4583670149937548076

Question: Can a physician be found liable for failing to inform a patient of the consequences of not getting a recommended medical test?

Answer: Yes.

Rena Truman was a 30-year-old woman who died after having been diagnosed with late stage cervical cancer. She had not had a Pap smear for 5 years despite regular visits to her family practitioner, Dr. Claude Thomas. Following her death, her two children sued Dr. Thomas for malpractice. At trial the judge refused to permit jury instruction that a physician has a duty to disclose all relevant information, including the risk of refusing procedures. The jury found in favor of Dr. Thomas, but upon appeal the Supreme Court of California reversed the trial court decision, citing judicial error. The court considered whether the physician breached his duty when he did not inform Mrs. Truman of the risk of failing to receive a Pap smear. Dr. Thomas contended that patients who reject their physician's advice should shoulder the burden of possible consequences. He also argued that he did not have a duty because the danger was remote and commonly known. The court explained that a patient is dependent on the physician for information because the physician has a greater degree of specialized medical knowledge. The court noted that despite being remote, the risk was death, and there was no evidence that the risk was commonly known. The court held that all material information that a reasonable person would want to know was relevant, including the risk of refusing a test.

CLITES V. IOWA, 322 N.W.2D 917 (1982)

Link to case: http://ia.findacase.com/research/wfrmDocViewer.aspx/xq/fac.19820629_0042174.IA.htm/qx

Question: Can failure to obtain informed consent for antipsychotic medication be grounds for malpractice?

Answer: Yes.

Timothy Clites was a man with mental retardation who was placed in restraints and received a variety of antipsychotic medications for aggressive behavior while admitted to a state-operated residential facility. Mr. Clites developed tardive dyskinesia after 5 years of treatment. His father sued for a violation of civil rights and damages from negligence. The trial court found for Mr. Clites, citing a lack of evidence of aggression, no regular evaluation by a physician for 3 years, no consultation for tardive dyskinesia, use of medications and restraints as a convenience, and lack of informed consent. The Iowa Court of Appeals affirmed the decision while clarifying informed consent required for administration of antipsychotic medication. The court reasoned that the concept of a right to privacy implied an underlying right to think and decide for oneself. Absent an emergency situation, a competent patient has a fundamental right to decide to be left alone without medications. The court concluded that there is a recognized standard that requires informed consent prior to administration of antipsychotic medication. As part of informed consent, a physician has a duty to make a reasonable disclosure of the nature and probable consequences of the recommended treatment.

ZINERMON V. BURCH, 494 U.S. 113 (1990)

Link to case: http://scholar.google.com/scholar_case?case=17065115765946990987

Question: Can an incompetent individual consent to voluntary hospitalization?

Answer: No.

Darrell Burch was admitted to a Florida state mental hospital in 1981 after being found wandering on a highway in Tallahassee while hallucinating, telling officials he was "in heaven." He signed voluntary admission forms despite never having been evaluated for capacity. Voluntary admission in Florida required "express and informed consent." He later brought a civil rights action claiming that the hospital had deprived him of liberty without due process as afforded by the Fourteenth Amendment. Mr. Burch alleged that state law was violated because the hospital should have known that he was incompetent to give informed consent to sign voluntary forms; hence he was entitled to procedural safeguards of an involuntary admission. The case was initially dismissed, but the U.S. Supreme Court ultimately agreed with Mr. Burch. It held that because the hospital's staff had authority to deprive persons of liberty, the Constitution imposed on them the state's duty to provide procedural protections. The Court contended that it was foreseeable that a person requesting treatment for mental illness might not be capable of informed consent, which should be specifically assessed at the time of admission. The state's violation of the duty to investigate the patient's competence was "fully predictable" and not a "random, unauthorized" violation of law as the state contended.

CHAPTER 3

Duty to Protect

ANDREW M. KOPELMAN

TARASOFF V. REGENTS, 551 P.2D 334 (1976)

Link to case: http://www.stanford.edu/group/psylawseminar/Tarsoff%20I.htm

Question: Is there a therapist duty to protect a third party from a dangerous patient?

Answer: Yes.

The parents of Tatiana Tarasoff sued the University of California and the psychologist working for its student health clinic after a patient in this clinic, Mr. Prosenjit Poddar, murdered Ms. Tarasoff. Mr. Poddar had confided to his psychologist his intention to kill Ms. Tarasoff, who was readily identifiable by Mr. Poddar's description. While the doctor and clinic did take some steps to contain the risk that Mr. Poddar represented, such as notifying the campus police, no one directly warned Ms. Tarasoff. The trial court found that the psychologist could not be held directly liable for failing to successfully hospitalize Mr. Poddar; the appeals court agreed, and a further appeal was made to the California Supreme Court. That court reversed the appellate decision in 1974 and found that therapists have a duty to *warn* individuals threatened by patients (known as *Tarasoff* I). In light of unusual protest about this decision, including from psychiatrists, the California Supreme Court agreed to hear the case again in 1976 (*Tarasoff* II). Beginning its analysis with the common law assumption that no one owed a duty to control the conduct of another, the court held that the special relationship between a psychotherapist and a patient created a duty to *protect* others from an identifiably dangerous patient based on the logic of foreseeability. The court majority relied heavily on precedents involving contagious diseases to formulate this notion. Once clinical circumstances established this duty, the psychotherapist was compelled to "exercise reasonable care" in protecting the potential victim, including possibly—but not necessarily—directly warning the potential victim. As the court maintained, "The protective privilege [i.e., confidentiality] ends where the public peril begins."

LIPARI V. SEARS, 497 F. SUPP. 1985 (1980)

Link to case: http://scholar.google.com/scholar_case?case=1021277736768084136

Question: Does a psychiatrist's duty to protect third parties extend to foreseeable, but unidentified, third parties?

Answer: Yes.

Ruth Ann Lipari sued Sears & Roebuck Co. after she was shot and her husband was killed by Ulysses Cribbs in a crowded nightclub in Omaha, Nebraska. Mr. Cribbs had purchased the shotgun at Sears. Mr. Cribbs had previously been committed to a Veterans Administration (VA) psychiatric hospital and subsequently treated as a VA outpatient approximately 1 month before the shooting. Mrs. Lipari argued that Sears should not have sold a gun to someone who was known to be "mentally defective." Sears in turn filed a third-party suit under the Federal Torts Claim Act, alleging that the VA hospital's negligent care of Mr. Cribbs was the proximate cause for the shooting injury and death. Mrs. Lipari then sued the U.S. government as well. The government petitioned the Nebraska Supreme Court for a summary motion dismissing these claims. In rejecting the government's position, the Nebraska court extended the reasoning of *Tarasoff* (California) to the state of Nebraska. The court affirmed that the special relationship between a psychotherapist and a patient imposed an affirmative duty to protect third parties from potentially dangerous patients. In acknowledging the technical difficulties related to violence prediction, the court explained that psychiatrists were not responsible for all acts of dangerous patients. Rather, the liability from a failure in the duty to protect arose from negligent practice that did not meet the professional standard of "due care." The victims need not be readily identifiable as was the case in *Tarasoff*, but instead belong to a "class of persons" who could be "reasonably foreseen" to be harmed by the dangerous patient.

PETERSEN V. WASHINGTON, 671 P.2D 230 (1983)

Link to case: http://www.leagle.com/decision/1983521100W n2d421_1482

Question: Does a psychiatrist's duty to third parties include protecting foreseeable victims from potential danger caused by a patient's noncompliance with medication?

Answer: Yes.

Cynthia Petersen sued the State of Washington after being injured in a motor vehicle accident involving a driver, Larry Knox, who ran a red light while under the influence of drugs. Mr. Knox had been released from a state psychiatric hospital only 5 days prior. Dr. Alva Miller, Mr. Knox's psychiatrist, argued that Mr. Knox had "recovered" at the time of his discharge. The trial court allowed rebuttal evidence about Mr. Knox's previous psychotic presentations to hospitals and subsequent arrests. A jury found that Dr. Miller negligently treated Mr. Knox by failing to seek further involuntary confinement at the time of discharge, and that this negligence was the proximate cause of Ms. Petersen injuries. On appeal, the Supreme Court of Washington affirmed the verdict, agreeing that the special relationship between a psychiatrist and a patient created a third-party duty to protect anyone who might "foreseeably be endangered" by Mr. Knox's illness, including his propensity to stop medication and return to abusing PCP. The court rejected the state's claim that it was not liable for negligence because Dr. Miller was performing a "discretionary activity of government" (i.e., performing an activity related to basic governmental policy) in completing a risk assessment.

JABLONSKI V. U.S., 712 F.2D 391 (1983)

Link to case: http://scholar.google.com/scholar_case?case=1021277736768084136

Question: Is a psychiatrist required to protect a foreseeable victim in the absence of a specific threat?

Answer: Yes.

Philip Jablonski received an outpatient evaluation at the Loma Linda VA hospital after threatening Melinda Kimball's mother. Diagnosing the patient with "anti-social personality," the psychiatrist, Dr. Kopiloff, did not make an effort to obtain Mr. Jablonski's medical records, which revealed the patient had suffered from schizophrenia and had tried to kill his previous wife on multiple occasions. Mr. Jablonski returned for another evaluation with Dr. Kopiloff's supervisor, but he was not hospitalized. Three days later he killed Ms. Kimball. Meghan Jablonski, Ms. Kimball's daughter, sued the U.S. government for malpractice, claiming that Dr. Kopiloff had not adequately incorporated information from the police into his assessment, had not pursued the patient's medical record, and had not specifically warned Ms. Kimball that she was at risk. The district court agreed. On appeal, the Ninth Circuit Court of Appeals affirmed the decision, rejecting the government's claim that the treating psychiatrist was subject to immunity under the Federal Torts Claim Act. The court also concluded that although Mr. Jablonski had never specifically voiced threats to Dr. Kopiloff related to Ms. Kimball, she could have been clearly identified and warned as the likely victim based on Mr. Jablonski's history of domestic abuse when psychotic in the past.

NAIDU V. LAIRD, 539 A.2D 1064 (1988)

Link to case: http://scholar.google.com/scholar_case?case=10922092048534834221

Question: Does a psychiatrist have a duty to protect the public from a dangerous former patient?

Answer: Yes.

Ann Laird sued Dr. Venkataramana Naidu of Delaware State Hospital (DSH) after Mrs. Laird's husband was killed in a motor vehicle accident caused by a recent patient of DSH, Hilton Putney. Mr. Putney had been discharged from DSH by Dr. Naidu 5 months prior after submitting a sign-out letter during a voluntary hospitalization. A jury found that Dr. Naidu's decision to discharge the patient without an adequate follow-up plan and without consideration of an involuntary commitment order was an act of negligence and the proximate cause of Mr. Laird's death. The Supreme Court of Delaware affirmed, first applying *Tarasoff* logic to affirm that the special relationship between Dr. Naidu and his patient created a third-party "broad-based obligation to protect the public from potentially violent patients." The court dismissed Dr. Naidu's claim that he was not obligated to consider Mr. Putney's psychiatric history in making an immediate assessment of dangerousness. Evidence presented at trial demonstrated that Dr. Naidu had not properly reviewed the extensive records from Mr. Putney's multiple prior hospitalizations demonstrating a history of poor medication compliance. In accepting the jury's finding of fact that Dr. Naidu's negligent decision was the proximate cause of Mr. Laird's death, the court also held that "temporal span" alone (i.e., more than 5 months since discharge) was not sufficient to absolve Dr. Naidu of responsibility. Finally, the court rejected Dr. Naidu's and the Delaware Psychiatric Association's arguments that the general inexactitude of dangerousness predictions prevented a case-by-case recovery from negligent psychiatric decision making, or that a verdict against Dr. Naidu might create destructive public policy in encouraging psychiatrists to avoid treating potentially violent patients or to overpredict dangerousness.

CHAPTER 4

Expert Testimony

SCOTT SOLOWAY AND BRYAN C. SHELBY

FRYE V. U.S., 293 F. 1013 (1923)

Link to case: http://www.law.ufl.edu/_pdf/faculty/little/topic8.pdf

Question: Is evidence acceptable in a federal criminal trial if not yet accepted by the scientific community?

Answer: No.

James Frye was convicted of murder. He appealed his conviction to the DC Circuit Court of Appeals, claiming that the lower court did not allow him to present results of the "systolic blood pressure deception test" he had undergone. His legal team argued that an expert "skilled in that particular science, art, or trade to which the question relates" could testify. The attorneys for Frye and the court recognized that no clear case law existed defining rules for the admissibility of scientific evidence. The court of appeals found that a given scientific principle, from which an expert's testimony is deduced, "must be sufficiently established to have gained general acceptance in the particular field." It ruled that "evidential force" lies somewhere between the "experimental" and "demonstrable" stages of scientific discovery. The lie detection test had not yet gained general acceptance, so the lower court's judgment was affirmed. Some states' courts (e.g., New York) still use this "Frye test" or "general acceptance" test to determine the admissibility of scientific expert testimony.

STATE V. HURD, 133 N.J. SUPER. 333 (1980)

Link to case: http://scholar.google.com/scholar_case?case=10872079423316724679

Question: Is hypnotically refreshed testimony of a crime victim that meets certain criteria reliable such that it is admissible in New Jersey courts?

Answer: Yes.

Jane Sell was sleeping in her apartment when an assailant attacked her. Afterward, she could not recollect the identity of her attacker. She underwent hypnosis at the suggestion of the prosecution to assist her recall. Under hypnosis, she identified her ex-husband, Paul Hurd, as the assailant. The defense moved to suppress her hypnotically refreshed testimony under the Fourteenth Amendment Due Process Clause. After considering the testimony from several experts, the trial court found that hypnotically refreshed testimony by a victim is admissible only on a case-by-case basis and that the state has the burden of proof by clear and convincing evidence to establish its reliability. Furthermore, in order to assure that the testimony is not coercive, the court adopted six standards for admissibility: (1) sessions must be conducted by a licensed psychiatrist or psychologist; (2) examiners involved must be independent; (3) information obtained by law enforcement should be written; (4) facts should be obtained from the subject before hypnosis; (5) sessions should be videotaped; and (6) only the hypnotist and the subject should be present during the session. The court held that the testimony presented in this case was inadmissible because it did not meet these standards.

PEOPLE V. SHIRLEY, 31 CAL. 3D 18 (1982)

Link to case: http://scholar.google.com/scholar_case?case=6644726564566919322

Question: In California, can a witness testify after using hypnosis to refresh his memory?

Answer: No.

Donald Shirley was accused of raping Catherine C., a woman who worked at a bar near Camp Pendleton in California. The consistent fact pattern of the crime involved Ms. C.'s intoxication and later sexual intercourse with Mr. Shirley. He asserted that the interaction was consensual and that he had been invited to Ms. C.'s apartment when he had met her in the bar hours prior. Ms. C. was unable to recall important details of the events and, on the eve of the trial, underwent hypnosis by a deputy district attorney with "some training" in the procedure. The trial court allowed this testimony over Mr. Shirley's objection that Ms. C.'s recollection of events under hypnosis was "manufactured evidence." There were significant differences in her pre- and posthypnosis testimony, although she was consistent in her report of at least some forced sexual activity. Dr. Donald Shafer was called by the defense as an expert on hypnosis and testified about its lack of reliability in this case. Despite this, Mr. Shirley was convicted. He appealed the decision to the Supreme Court of California. That court agreed with him and reversed the trial court finding, ruling that even the safeguards outlined in *State v. Hurd* were not enough to overcome the lack of reliability of hypnotically refreshed testimony. It found that this form of evidence did not meet the *Frye* standard of general acceptance in the scientific community and was therefore inadmissible.

ROCK V. ARKANSAS, 483 U.S. 44 (1987)

Link to case: http://scholar.google.com/scholar_case?case=4171699802405503521

Question: Does Arkansas's blanket rule barring all hypnotically refreshed testimony by a defendant violate one's constitutional right to testify on one's own behalf?

Answer: Yes.

Vickie Lorene Rock was charged with manslaughter in the death of her husband, who was found shot with a bullet wound to his chest. Ms. Rock was not able to remember the exact details of the shooting, and at the request of her attorney, she underwent hypnosis to refresh her recollection of those events. Under hypnosis, she related details of the shooting, including the assertion that she had not intentionally fired the gun. These details were supported by the testimony of a firearms expert. Ms. Rock's testimony, however, was excluded because Arkansas had a per se rule excluding the admission of a criminal defendant's hypnotically refreshed testimony. On appeal, the U.S. Supreme Court held that an absolute prohibition of hypnotically refreshed testimony violates Fifth, Sixth, and Fourteenth Amendment rights. Specifically, it violates the right to be heard, the right to confront witnesses, and the right to testify on one's own behalf. The Court ruled that admissibility of such testimony should be admitted on a case-by-case basis and cannot be barred by a blanket rule.

DAUBERT V. MERRELL DOW PHARMACEUTICALS, 509 U.S. 579 (1993)

Link to case: http://caselaw.lp.findlaw.com/scripts/getcase.pl?navby=case&court=us&vol=509&page=579

Question: Is *Frye* v. *U.S.* the appropriate standard for admitting scientific evidence into a federal court?

Answer: No.

Jason Daubert and Eric Schuller, minor children, and their parents sued Merrell Dow pharmaceuticals for serious birth defects they alleged were caused by the mothers' taking of the antinausea medication Bendectin. Dow's expert opined that, based on all published studies, the drug was not teratogenic in humans. Daubert and others presented eight experts who, based on "reanalysis" of studies, opined that the drug could be teratogenic. Both the district court and the U.S. Court of Appeals for the Ninth Circuit found that the eight experts' testimonies did not meet the *Frye* test. On appeal, the U.S. Supreme Court unanimously found that the *Frye* test had been superseded by the Federal Rules of Evidence (first enacted in 1975). The majority of justices agreed that these rules require the trial judge to determine, through an assessment of an expert's evidence, that expert testimony "rests on a reliable foundation" and is "relevant" to understanding or determining an issue at hand. The Court offered a list of guidelines for admissibility of scientific testimony that focus on the methods, rather than the conclusions, of an expert's evidence. These guidelines are as follows: (1) Are the methods and/or rationale scientifically valid? (2) Has the theory been subject to peer review or publication? (3) Can or has the theory been tested? (4) What is the theory's or technique's known or potential error rate? (5) Are there standards that relate to the technique? (6) Is there widespread acceptance of the technique in the scientific community?

GENERAL ELECTRIC V. JOINER, 522 U.S. 136 (1997)

Link to case: http://caselaw.lp.findlaw.com/scripts/getcase.pl?navby=case&court=us&vol=522&page=136

Question: Should an appellate court use the "abuse of discretion" standard in reviewing a trial court's decision to admit or exclude expert testimony?

Answer: Yes.

Robert Joiner claimed that his work exposed him to hazardous PCBs and their derivatives and that such exposure "promoted" his developing lung cancer. The District Court in Georgia granted summary judgment for General Electric based in part on the failure of Mr. Joiner's experts to show a link between PCBs and small-cell lung cancer. The judge found that the referenced animal and human studies either were not sufficiently relevant to Mr. Joiner's circumstances or were misinterpreted by Mr. Joiner's experts to bolster his claims. The court found that the expert opinion was speculative and *ipse dixit* (just because the expert said it was true). The U.S. Court of Appeals for the Eleventh Circuit reversed this decision, finding that the district court had overstepped its role by ruling on conclusions of experts rather than the "legal reliability" of evidence. The U.S. Supreme Court then reversed the court of appeals, unanimously agreeing that "abuse of discretion" (a judge's failure to properly consider a fact or law) is the appropriate standard for appellate review and that the district court had properly considered these issues.

KUMHO TIRE CO. V. CARMICHAEL, 526 U.S. 137 (1999)

Link to case: http://scholar.google.com/scholar_case?case=11404623739922196630

Question: Does the *Daubert* decision apply to testimony from engineers and nonscientific testimony?

Answer: Yes.

Patrick Carmichael claimed that the minivan he was driving had a defective tire, made by Kumho Tire Co., that blew out and caused a motor vehicle accident that led to the death of one of the passengers and severe injury to others. He relied heavily on the expert opinion of a tire failure analyst, Dennis Carlson Jr. The district court found initially and again on review that key technical evidence was not admissible under *Daubert* because it did not meet the reliability standards (e.g., scientifically reliable methodology, subject to peer review, known error rate) established in that case. The U.S. Court of Appeals for the Eleventh Circuit reversed the decision and remanded it for further consideration, stating that the district court should not have applied a "*Daubert* analysis" to a case that did not involve scientific evidence. The U.S. Supreme Court subsequently reversed the appellate decision and put to rest any doubt that *Daubert* applied to all expert testimony; all expert evidence is subject to judicial gatekeeping. The Court wrote that trial judges might apply the factors recommended by *Daubert* for reviewing scientific evidence to nonscientific evidence.

CHAPTER 5

Questions on Mental Health Practice Guidelines

QUESTIONS

1. In order to pass the "*Frye* test," experts must be able to:
   A. Show that their peers have accepted the science used in testimony
   B. Present scientific evidence to the court in support of their testimony
   C. Demonstrate their scientific tests in court
   D. Present published papers or books that support their opinion
   E. Present their own publications supporting their opinions

2. In multiple appellate court decisions, the broadest guiding principal limiting a psychiatrist's duty to protect a third party from a dangerous patient has been formulated as follows:
   A. Only when the name of a specific potential victim is identified does a psychiatrist incur a duty to protect.
   B. Only when a specific potential victim is identified does a psychiatrist incur a duty to protect.
   C. Only when a specific threat is made in the presence of the psychiatrist is a duty incurred.
   D. A psychiatrist has a duty to protect any class of persons who may be foreseeably harmed by a dangerous patient.

3. Hypnotically refreshed testimony may have usefulness:
   A. In guaranteeing the truth of repressed memory
   B. In accurately relaying very specific forgotten details

C. In helping a subject relax and concentrate in order to better relay information
D. In avoiding coerced testimony

4. "Abuse of discretion" in the context of the law means:
   A. A judge inappropriately applies the law.
   B. A judge abuses his or her discretion in evaluating evidence for admission.
   C. A judge decides arbitrarily or blatantly in error about evidentiary admissibility.
   D. All of the above.

5. It is more difficult to obtain adequate informed consent for experiments with involuntarily committed patients because:
   A. A high risk-to-benefit ratio requires greater understanding.
   B. Involuntarily committed patients may not be as informed.
   C. A lack of liberty requires procedural protections regarding informed consent.
   D. Involuntarily committed patients may have less monitoring.
   E. Involuntarily confined patients live in an "inherently coercive" environment, which might make it difficult for them to voluntarily consent.

6. The *Daubert* majority recommends that the judge conducting a preliminary *Daubert* hearing inquire about:
   A. Whether the science has been tested
   B. Whether the science has been peer reviewed and published
   C. Whether the science has a known or potential rate of error
   D. Whether the science has been generally accepted
   E. All of the above

7. The legal standard outlining a psychiatrist's duty to protect others from a potentially dangerous patient:
   A. Has been established at a federal level by a U.S. Supreme Court decision
   B. Has been established as a federal law by act of Congress
   C. Has developed from state-specific case law that is binding only at a state level
   D. Was first outlined and advocated by the American Psychiatric Association

8. Hypnotically refreshed testimony:
   A. Is equivalent in reliability to a test for blood-type

B. Has well-established validity
C. Is treated the same in virtually all jurisdictions
D. Is available only in cases involving homicide crimes
E. Has the potential to be unreliable

9. Under *Frye*, a psychiatric expert's testimony that contradicted a statement in the *Diagnostic and Statistical Manual of Mental Disorders* (*DSM*) would be most problematic if that expert had testified that the *DSM* is:
   A. Instructive
   B. Commonly used
   C. Written by experts in the field
   D. Authoritative
   E. Merely a guide in formulating a diagnosis

10. You have been treating a woman in your private practice for the past 5 years. She is a 69-year-old retired widow who lives with her son. During your session, you notice that she has a black eye covered with makeup and bruises on her arms. During therapy, she breaks down crying and divulges that her son has been beating her up. She begs you not to say anything to the authorities because she feels that she is financially dependent on her son and scared to live alone. What is the most appropriate way to handle this confidentiality situation?
    A. Reassure her that you will maintain confidentiality and provide her with a pamphlet of community support resources for battered women.
    B. Validate her fears and reassure her that HIPPA laws prohibit you from sharing any unauthorized clinical information.
    C. Invite the son to her next therapy appointment to work through conflicts that may be occurring in the home.
    D. Validate her fears but inform her that this is a case of elder abuse and you need to report this abuse to the authorities for her safety.
    E. Inform her that as a psychiatrist, you are required to maintain her confidentiality. However, you will inform her internist, who may decide to report the abuse to the authorities.

11. As a result of the *Daubert, Joiner,* and *Kumho Tire* decisions, Rule 702 of the Federal Rules of Evidence has been amended to include which condition for admissibility of expert testimony?
    A. The expert's knowledge is limited to information based only on academic work and not on experience.

B. Testimony is based on precedent from relevant case law.
C. Testimony is the product of reliable principles and methods.
D. The expert received training at a reputable medical school.

12. Privilege belongs to:
    A. The patient's defense attorney
    B. The prosecuting attorney
    C. The patient's treating clinician
    D. The patient
    E. The patient's next of kin

13. Modern informed consent decisions are primarily driven by the concept of:
    A. Autonomy
    B. Paternalism
    C. Justice
    D. Beneficence
    E. Competence

14. A mental health expert's concerns about the future of mental health testimony under the *Daubert* standard might include:
    A. Likelihood of "junk" science being admitted into evidence
    B. Role of the judge as gatekeeper
    C. A judge's reticence to admit a complicated but generally accepted psychological test
    D. All of the above

15. In federal courts, hypnotically refreshed testimony offered by defendants is:
    A. Inadmissible absent a showing of undue hardship
    B. Admissible subject to the Federal Rules of Evidence
    C. Admissible under the *Frye* standard
    D. Inadmissible under the *Daubert* standard

16. In *Naidu v. Laird*, the Delaware Supreme Court agreed that Dr. Naidu's decision to discharge a psychiatric patient was the proximate cause of Mr. Laird's death because:
    A. The patient was discharged the same day his psychotic behavior led to Mr. Laird's death.
    B. The patient was discharged only a month before his psychotic behavior led to Mr. Laird's death.
    C. The court found that temporal span alone was not a sole determination of proximate cause.
    D. None of the above.

17. A man with chronic schizophrenia is evaluated in the emergency room and appears to be actively hallucinating. He says that he wants to sign himself into the hospital because the aliens tell him to do so. As a psychiatrist you should:
    A. Allow the patient to voluntarily sign himself into the hospital.
    B. Sign the patient into the hospital as an involuntary patient.
    C. Assess for competence to sign voluntary admission forms and allow him to sign if competent.
    D. If not competent to sign voluntary papers, sign the patient into the hospital as an involuntary patient based only on his lack of competence.

18. As outlined in *Tarasoff*, the duty of a psychiatrist to protect a third party from a potentially dangerous patient:
    A. Is based on a psychotherapist's responsibility for his or her patient's actions as part of the legal treatment framework
    B. Arises from abilities psychiatrists are supposed to have to predict violence in the mentally ill
    C. Arises purely from a functional policy directive intended to minimize violent behavior in the mentally ill
    D. Is rooted in the special relationship between a psychotherapist and a patient, with an emphasis on foreseeability

19. Which of the following was a safeguard to ensure reliability of hypnotically refreshed testimony as established in *State v. Hurd*?
    A. Sessions should be conducted by a licensed psychiatrist or psychologist.
    B. The hypnotist should be independent of the parties involved.
    C. Sessions should be videotaped.
    D. Only the hypnotist and the subject should present during the session.
    E. All of the above.

20. Which of the following best explains the scope of the relationship between physician–patient privilege and group therapy?
    A. Physician–patient privilege does not extend to group therapy because patients waive their confidentiality rights when they agree to participate in a group therapy format, which by nature requires open disclosure.
    B. Physician–patient privilege supersedes mandated reporting of child abuse if the perpetrator is engaged in mental health treatment.

C. Mandated reporting of child abuse rarely preempts physician–patient privilege.
D. The Federal Comprehensive Alcohol Abuse and Alcoholism Prevention, Treatment and Rehabilitation Act Amendments of 1974 included provisions to protect a patient's identity, diagnosis, prognosis, and treatment and preempts the state's mandated reporting requirements.
E. Federal laws designed to protect the identity, diagnosis, prognosis, and treatment of patients engaged in alcohol or drug treatment are preempted by state-mandated reporting of child abuse requirements.

21. Informed consent must be:
    A. Voluntary
    B. Informed
    C. Competent
    D. All of the above

22. Which of the following is true regarding mandated reporting requirements?
    A. They include requirements to provide referrals and treatment to appropriate aftercare services.
    B. Physicians and psychologists are required to provide informed consent on evidence-based, trauma-focused cognitive behavioral therapy.
    C. They are jurisdiction dependent.
    D. They represent a discretionary duty for professionals.

23. Informed consent is required in which of the following situations?
    A. Before prescribing standing antipsychotic medications
    B. Before seclusion in the hospital
    C. Before administering an emergency intramuscular injection for dangerousness
    D. When the patient is admitted to a hospital involuntarily

24. The *Kumho Tire* opinion suggests that expert testimony based on clinical experience would be:
    A. Inadmissible on its face
    B. More highly scrutinized than scientific or technical expert testimony
    C. Admissible only when there is proof that it is scientific

D. Subject to the same inquiry to assure reliability and relevance as other testimony
E. Exempt from *Daubert*

25. Various state appellate courts have found which of the following as evidence of negligence in failing to exercise reasonable care to discharge the duty to protect third persons from a potentially dangerous patient?
    A. Failing to adequately review records related to a patient's past psychiatric history prior to discharging the patient.
    B. Failing to consider involuntarily hospitalizing a voluntary patient, and agreeing to discharge him instead without a reasonable aftercare plan.
    C. Failing to address a patient's likelihood of relapsing on drugs of abuse and not taking prescribed medication after discharge.
    D. All of the above.

26. The following statement best reflects the rationale for the ruling in *State v. Andring*:
    A. A patient's self-incriminating statements made during group therapy are different than those made during individual therapy and are therefore admissible to a court of law.
    B. The standard of confidentiality that protects physician–patient privilege during testimony in a trial is different than the standard for cooperating with law enforcement during an investigation of sexual abuse.
    C. Mental health treatment records are not considered to be protected by physician–patient privilege.
    D. Group therapy treatment records are protected by physician–patient confidentiality.
    E. When alleged perpetrators are enrolled in sexual offender treatment, they waive their right to confidentiality.

27. What is the significance of the following statement from the majority's decision in *Tarasoff*: "The protective privilege ends where the public peril begins"?
    A. A psychiatrist's duty to protect others from a dangerous patient is ultimately limited by public policy arguments protecting the confidential nature of the doctor–patient relationship.
    B. A psychiatrist's duty to protect the confidential nature of communications with a patient is ultimately limited by the need to protect the public from a potential and foreseeable danger.

C. A psychiatrist's responsibility to the public is ultimately greater than his responsibility to keep one particular patient safe.
D. A psychiatrist must protect his privilege to practice his profession but must also keep the public safe from psychiatric overclaim.

28. In which situation would a physician not have to give information regarding the risk of refusing a procedure?
    A. If the patient is a physician
    B. If the risk is commonly known
    C. If the risk is very rare
    D. If the patient is signing him- or herself in voluntarily to a hospital

ANSWERS

1. **A**

    The lower court denied *Frye*'s expert an opportunity to demonstrate the systolic blood pressure deception test in court, a denial affirmed by the appellate court. The court ruled that general acceptance of experts would determine whether this deception test could be accepted as scientifically sound. While presenting evidence from one's own research or that of peers might be useful, it is the general acceptance by the scientific community of one's opinions that is essential.

2. **D**

    Although state courts have varied in their definition of foreseeable victims, courts have found that psychiatrists are liable for failing to protect foreseeable victims when the name of the victim was not known (*Tarasoff v. Regents*), when no specific victim was threatened (*Naidu v. Laird* and *Lipari v. Sears*), and when no specific threat was made to the psychiatrist (*Jablonski v. U.S.*). The broadest formulation of the limits of a psychiatrist's duty to protect is that he or she take reasonable care to protect all foreseeable victims from a patient clinically judged to represent a danger to others.

3. **C**

    Despite the potential for hypnotically refreshed testimony to be unreliable, it has established usefulness in helping witnesses become more relaxed and to concentrate. Hypnosis does have the potential for coercion, and hypnotically refreshed testimony does not guarantee truth or the accuracy of details.

QUESTIONS ON MENTAL HEALTH PRACTICE GUIDELINES (33)

4. **D**

"Abuse of discretion" is a term of art that refers to judicial inappropriateness in considering a law or a fact. Judges are given discretion in making all sorts of decisions, including the admissibility of evidence. "Abuse of discretion" commonly refers to the standard an appeals court must apply in reviewing a lower court's decision regarding what evidence was admitted at trial.

5. **E**

In *Kaimowitz v. Department of Mental Health for the State of Michigan*, the court ruled that involuntarily confined patients were unable to give consent for experimental psychosurgery. The court reasoned that a lack of liberty as related to involuntary commitment created an inherently coercive environment that made it more difficult to obtain adequate voluntary informed consent (E). A lack of liberty requiring greater procedural protections in informed consent is a general concept (C) but is not as specific an answer in describing why it is difficult to obtain informed consent for experimental research on involuntarily committed patients. A high risk-to-benefit ratio would require a greater level of understanding for informed consent but is not unique to involuntarily committed patients (A). Involuntarily committed patients could be as informed (B) and have equal monitoring (D) as other patients and does not explain the core difficulty of obtaining adequate informed consent for this group.

6. **E**

The Court gives some guidance regarding what the trial judge at a preliminary hearing might use to assess admissibility of evidence. The Court relies on scientific publications in suggesting these considerations. The majority demotes the *Frye* "standard" to merely a consideration; evidence not generally accepted "may properly be viewed with skepticism."

7. **C**

The legal standard outlining a psychiatrist's duty to protect others from a potentially dangerous patient was first elucidated in the majority opinion of the California Supreme Court in *Tarasoff v. Regents* in 1976. Multiple subsequent appellate courts in various states have since found similarly in state-specific cases, but there is no U.S. Supreme Court precedent or national statute instituting a duty to protect on a federal level. The APA filed an amicus brief arguing against imposing such a duty on psychotherapists in *Tarasoff*.

8. **E**

   While hypnotically refreshed testimony is admissible, it does not have the same reliability status as a blood test. There is controversy around its use and validity, but courts have the option to adopt safeguards and guidelines as was done in *State v. Hurd* to ensure reliability as applied in a particular case. These guidelines do not have to be identical for all states. Although the two cases described, *Rock v. Arkansas* and *State v. Hurd*, involved homicide, hypnotically refreshed testimony is not limited to cases involving homicide.

9. **D**

   Because the *Frye* test is the "general acceptance" test, the more generally accepted a piece of evidence, the less reliable any expert testimony that contradicts that piece of evidence would be. Once the expert has stated that a given text is authoritative, any evidence to the contrary would be less likely to pass muster under the *Frye* standard. Other descriptors that emphasize the limits of the *DSM* on a given issue (and, of course, other "generally accepted" evidence) would be more conducive to gaining the admissibility of an expert's statements that contradict the *DSM*.

10. **D**

    In this case, you have an obligation to address the woman's abusive situation. The laws about reporting elder abuse (and child abuse) allow you to break confidentiality and report suspected abuse. Simply giving the patient a pamphlet is an insufficient intervention to protect her. HIPAA laws do not prohibit a clinician from reporting elder abuse. Inviting her son to her therapy session to address his abusive behavior would not be an appropriate intervention and would be insufficient to protect this patient. Passing this information on to her internist without reporting would not fulfill the required duty.

11. **C**

    The Federal Rules of Evidence were amended in 2000 and again in 2011 to incorporate the *Daubert* decision and its so-called progeny. These amendments indicate the permanence in the shift toward judicial gatekeeping and scrutiny of expert testimony. Of the available choices, only C is correct. Expert knowledge can be based on relevant experience, case law is not considered a legitimate source of reliability for scientific evidence, and expert testimony does not have to be delivered by a medical doctor, much less one who trained at a reputable medical school.

12. **D**

    Privilege is the patient's right to bar the clinician from testifying about professionally obtained material in judicial or quasi-judicial settings (trials, depositions, hearings, etc.). A useful mnemonic is "P = Privilege = Patient."

13. **A**

    Paternalism relates to a right of the government to make policies to limit an individual's rights or liberties for the individual's own good. Paternalism is at odds with autonomy that relates to an individual's right to self-determination. Modern informed consent decisions have progressed from *Natanson v. Kline* to *Canterbury v. Spence* to *Truman v. Thomas* have moved away from paternalism (B) toward autonomy (A) as the driving concept behind their decisions. Justice is the fair treatment of individuals in a society (C). Beneficence is to do well to others (D). Neither is the driving concept behind informed consent decisions. An individual has to be competent (E) to give informed consent, but competence has not been used as an argument for informed consent.

14. **D**

    These concerns (and more) have been extensively discussed in forums and publications since the *Daubert* decision. Fears about an inevitable "*Daubert* challenge" are common, and many papers address the potential or actual *Daubert* challenges and results when psychiatric issues, particularly novel concepts or tests, are at issue. *Daubert* can present the mental health expert with obstacles, but it can also provide an opportunity for the expert to define and clarify the scientific basis of his or her testimony.

15. **B**

    Although the *Rock v. Arkansas* decision involved a state court issue, its holding involved basic constitutional rights, was decided by the U.S. Supreme Court, and is therefore applicable in federal courts. Thus, the Federal Rules of Evidence will govern the admissibility of any offered hypnotically refreshed testimony by a defendant. The *Daubert* criteria were incorporated into the Federal Rules of Evidence and do not automatically make hypnotically refreshed testimony inadmissible. Although the *Frye* opinion was a decision about expert testimony, it is no longer applicable in federal courts following the *Daubert* decision. "Undue hardship" is not a standard for hypnotically refreshed testimony admissibility.

16. **C**

    More than 5 months after Mr. Putney was discharged from the Delaware State Hospital and while he was still psychotic, he intentionally drove his car into Mr. Laird's car, killing Mr. Laird. The trial court found Mr. Putney's negligent discharge as the proximate cause of Mr. Laird's death. The Delaware Supreme Court agreed, refuting the argument that too much time had elapsed to link the psychiatric discharge to the cause of death. As the court noted, "temporal span" by itself was insufficient to define proximate causation.

17. **C**

In *Zinermon v. Burch*, the U.S. Supreme Court decided that it was foreseeable that a person requesting treatment for mental illness may not be competent to give informed consent for voluntary hospitalization, which should be specifically assessed at the time of admission. As such, patients should not be automatically able to voluntarily sign themselves into a hospital without a competence evaluation (A). Involuntary commitment criteria involve dangerousness *and* incompetence, not solely incompetence. A patient may not meet involuntary criteria (B), even if found incompetent to sign voluntary papers (D). In this situation the correct procedure would be (C), where the patient should be evaluated for competence to sign voluntary admission forms and, if competent, be allowed to sign.

18. **D**

The court in *Tarasoff* and other appellate courts have rooted the duty of a psychiatrist to protect a third party from a potentially dangerous patient in the special relationship between a psychotherapist and patient. This relationship puts a psychiatrist in a unique place to potentially foresee a danger to a particular third party or class of people, and in turn creates a duty to protect them. This duty is akin to that which a medical doctor has to the public when treating a potentially contagious patient. While the courts have acknowledged this duty, they have also voiced skepticism about psychiatry's actual ability to predict violence based on any scientific model. The duty arises in relation to specific foreseeable dangers; psychiatrists are otherwise not legally responsible for all of the conduct of their patients.

19. **E**

All of the choices presented in this question are safeguards that were presented in the *State v. Hurd* decision to help ensure reliability of hypnotically refreshed testimony. They were (1) sessions should be conducted by a licensed psychiatrist or psychologist; (2) parties involved should be independent; (3) information obtained by law enforcement should be written; (4) facts should be obtained from the subject before hypnosis; (5) sessions should be videotaped; and (6) only the hypnotist and subject should be present during the session.

20. **E**

    Federal laws designed to protect the identity, diagnosis, prognosis, and treatment of patients engaged in alcohol or drug treatment are preempted by state-mandated reporting of child abuse requirements. While the Federal Comprehensive Alcohol Abuse and Alcoholism Prevention, Treatment and Rehabilitation Act Amendments of 1974 included provisions to protect a patient's identity, diagnosis, prognosis, and treatment, the court ruled that this act did not preempt child abuse reporting requirements. The perpetrator's engagement in mental health treatment is not relevant to reporting reasonable suspicions of abuse. It is false to state that mandated reporting of child abuse rarely preempts physician–patient privilege; this type of reporting is an explicit exception to that privilege.

21. **D**

    Informed consent must involve each of the listed concepts (E). Informed consent must be voluntary (A) and free from coercion and duress. Problems with voluntariness arose in *Kaimowitz v. Department of Mental Health for the State of Michigan* where involuntarily committed patients were thought to be susceptible to coercion as related to their loss of liberty as involuntary patients. Informed consent must be informed (B), the amount of information having developed through case law in *Natanson v. Kline, Canterbury v. Spence*, and *Truman v. Thomas*. Finally, informed consent must be competent, and consent obtained when a patient is not competent may not be valid (C). In *Zinermon v. Burch* it was decided that incompetent individuals could not give informed consent for voluntary hospitalization.

22. **C**

    Mandated reporting requirements are jurisdiction dependent. They do not relate to duty to protect, and they do not require the mandated reporter to provide treatment referrals or aftercare services.

23. **A**

    Clites v. Iowa found that informed consent was required prior to administration of antipsychotic medication. *Zinermon v. Burch* found that informed consent was required to sign voluntary paperwork, which should be assessed at the time of hospital admission; however, involuntary hospital commitment typically implies a lack of capacity and therefore does not required informed consent. Seclusion and emergency intramuscular injections are considered emergency situations for a patient who is an acute danger to self and others and would be considered exceptions to the informed consent requirement as described in *Canterbury v. Spence*.

24. **D**

    According to the decision in *Daubert*, the role of judge as gatekeeper exists "to make certain that an expert, whether basing testimony upon professional studies or personal experience, employs in the courtroom the same level of intellectual rigor that characterizes the practice of an expert in the relevant field." *Daubert* factors can be applied to expert testimony, including psychiatric testimony, based on clinical experience and study. The U.S. Supreme Court in *Kumho Tire* stated that "a trial court should consider the specific factors identified in *Daubert* where there are reasonable measures of reliability of expert testimony."

25. **D**

    All of the choices have been found as evidence of negligence to discharge a duty to protect (*Jablonski v. U.S.*, *Naidu v. Laird*, and *Petersen v. Washington*). Rather than proscribe a specific set of universal actions necessary to discharge this duty, courts have consistently found that a psychiatrist need only follow a standard of care that a reasonable psychiatrist would pursue in a similar clinical situation to protect a potential third-party victim from a foreseeable danger.

26. **D**

    In *State v. Andring*, the court recognized that group therapy was no different than other forms of mental health treatment and, accordingly, was subject to the same levels of physician– patient confidentiality. Mental health treatment and group therapy records are both protected by physician–patient privilege. Physicians are included in the group of mandated reporters of child abuse, and this standard does not address physician–patient privilege or cooperation with law enforcement during an investigation of sexual abuse. Patients are entitled to physician–patient confidentiality regardless of the type of treatment in which they are engaged.

27. **B**

    When courts first outlined the scope of a psychiatrist's duty to protect third parties from foreseeable harm, many advocates of psychiatric treatment, including the APA, argued that compromising the confidential nature of the communication between a patient and a treating mental health clinician would jeopardize the very efficacy of treatment itself. However, various state appellate courts have consistently held that this privilege of confidential communication is not without limits and ultimately may be sacrificed when a foreseeable harm can be averted by breaking confidentiality.

28. **C**

Truman v. Thomas found that it constituted malpractice for a physician to fail to inform his or her patient of the consequences of refusing a medical procedure. Exceptions to disclosure include if the patient already knows the risk, such as if it is commonly known (e.g., getting sleepy from cough medicine). A rare risk (C) is not necessarily considered an exception because the risk could be significant, such as death, and be part of what a reasonable person would want to know.

SECTION II

Institutional Treatment Guidelines

This section highlights cases that relate to the confinement of individuals in hospital settings and the decisions with which they may be faced while hospitalized. Although many of the cases revolve around involuntary psychiatric treatment, included are cases about refusing medical care, including lifesaving interventions. Almost all of the cases involve the tension between paternalism (parens patriae), police power, and individual patient autonomy. While state jurisdictions may vary in terms of the specific application of the law, some national themes have emerged. For example, mental illness and dangerousness (despite being variably defined) are nationally accepted requirements for civil commitment, and patients who are involuntarily hospitalized are no longer considered incapable of making decisions. State jurisdictions also vary in the substantive standards for treating patients over their objection, varying from a rights-driven standard in Massachusetts to a treatment-focused approached in New Jersey.

Correctional institutions (e.g., jails and prisons) are not included in this section, although they are clearly institutions to which individuals are involuntarily confined and are considered under a similar umbrella as hospitals in the Civil Rights of Institutionalized Persons Act of 1980 (CRIPA). We have chosen instead to group all of the cases involving prisoners in the "Criminal Law and Incarceration" section. Although the cases raise issues that could also fit within other chapters (e.g., a prisoner's right to and right to refuse treatment), the broader class of "prisoners" more easily distinguishes this group.

CHAPTER 6

Civil Commitment

ELIZABETH FORD

LAKE V. CAMERON, 364 F.2D 657 (1966)

Link to case: http://scholar.google.com/scholar_case?case=16374362071956566586

Question: Can a civilly committed patient be involuntarily held in a hospital if there are safe, less restrictive treatment alternatives available?

Answer: No.

Catherine Lake, a 60-year-old woman, was found wandering around the streets of Washington, DC. She was picked up by two policemen and taken to DC General Hospital. She filed for a writ of habeas corpus in the DC Circuit Court and was transferred to St. Elizabeth's Hospital (where Dale Cameron was the superintendent) to await her civil commitment hearing. Her petition was denied without a hearing. In the meantime, the District of Columbia passed the Hospitalization of the Mentally Ill Act, allowing individuals with mental illness who are dangerous to themselves or others to be either hospitalized or treated in a manner that maintains their best interests and protects public safety. At Ms. Lake's subsequent commitment hearing, the examining psychiatrists found her to be of "unsound mind" and suffering from mild dementia. She appealed to the U.S. Court of Appeals, DC Circuit, which ruled that inpatient hospitalization was not necessarily the least restrictive alternative or the most appropriate for Ms. Lake, and the court held that the state had the obligation to explore these less restrictive alternatives when considering involuntary hospitalization for a patient. The court opined about the balance that might be obtained from protecting Ms. Lake's liberty interests by enlisting family or community services to keep her safe. It wrote, "Deprivations of liberty solely because of dangers to the ill persons themselves should not go beyond what is necessary for their protection."

BAXSTROM V. HEROLD, 383 U.S. 107 (1966)

Link to case: http://scholar.google.com/scholar_case?case=17820943305043602552

Question: Can an individual being released from prison be civilly committed without being afforded the right to a jury determination of such commitment?

Answer: No.

Johnnie Baxstrom had been incarcerated at a New York prison on an assault conviction for some months when he was certified as "insane." He was subsequently transferred to Dannemora State Hospital, operated by the New York Department of Correction. At the termination of his criminal sentence, two physicians and Dr. Herold certified at surrogate court that Mr. Baxstrom should be civilly committed and transferred to the custody of the New York Department of Mental Hygiene (DMH). However, the DMH did not think that Mr. Baxstrom was appropriate for their care system, and he therefore remained at Dannemora for more than 4 years after the completion of his criminal sentence. Mr. Baxstrom filed a writ of habeas corpus that he should be transferred to a civil facility if he was actually insane. The writ was denied several times by a state court and again by the Court of Appeals for New York. The U.S. Supreme Court granted certiorari and found that Mr. Baxstrom had been denied equal protection under the Fourteenth Amendment because he had been denied the right to jury review of the finding that he was mentally ill as is afforded all others who are facing civil commitment. The court did not find persuasive the state's argument that individuals evaluated for civil commitment at the end of penal sentences are categorically different than all others.

LESSARD V. SCHMIDT, 349 F. SUPP. 1078 (1972)

Link to case: http://scholar.google.com/scholar_case?case=16374362071956566586

Question: Should individuals facing civil commitment proceedings be entitled to due process rights similar to those in criminal proceedings?

Answer: Yes.

Alberta Lessard was brought to a mental health center in Milwaukee by two police officers. An emergency detention form was filed in order to detain her in the hospital. Three days later, with evidence presented from the officers related only to the initial reason for detention, the judge ordered a further 10 days of detention. At a subsequent hearing, upon petition of the mental health center claiming that Ms. Lessard should be "permanently committed" as a result of her schizophrenia, the judge ordered additional detention time. Ms. Lessard was not informed of any of these hearings or decisions. She filed a class action lawsuit in district court on behalf of herself and all involuntarily committed adults arguing that Wisconsin's involuntary commitment statute violated her due process rights. The court ruled in favor of Ms. Lessard, reasoning that because involuntary hospitalization was a significant deprivation of liberty in civil commitment hearings, the state was required to prove mental illness and dangerousness beyond a reasonable doubt and to ensure that less restrictive alternatives are not available. It also ruled that due process required that patients be given timely notice of their rights and have the right to legal counsel.

O'CONNOR V. DONALDSON, 422 U.S. 563 (1975)

Link to case: http://scholar.google.com/scholar_case?case=16877644373401713395

Question: Can a mentally ill patient be involuntarily committed to a hospital if he or she is not dangerous?

Answer: No.

Kenneth Donaldson had schizophrenia and was committed by his father under a relatively vague involuntary commitment statute to Florida State Hospital in Chattahoochee. While in the hospital for approximately 15 years, he was treated with "milieu therapy" but little else by way of therapy or medication. He did not behave in a manner that was dangerous to himself or others. Mr. Donaldson requested meetings with the superintendent of the hospital, Dr. J. B. O'Connor, as well as discharge, but was always denied. There were multiple people and organizations in the community willing to care for Mr. Donaldson. Dr. O'Connor eventually retired, Mr. Donaldson was released, and he filed suit, claiming that his constitutional right to liberty had been violated without providing required treatment. The district court and the U.S. Court of Appeals for the Fifth Circuit both found in favor of Mr. Donaldson and that he had a right to treatment as part of the Fourteenth Amendment. The U.S. Supreme Court heard the case but did not address the right to treatment issue. Instead, it found Mr. Donaldson's confinement unconstitutional because "a State cannot constitutionally confine without more a non-dangerous individual who is capable of surviving safely in freedom by himself or with the help of willing and responsible family members or friends."

ADDINGTON V. TEXAS, 441 U.S. 418 (1979)

Link to case: http://scholar.google.com/scholar_case?case=1383560548954406906

Question: Is "clear and convincing evidence" the burden of proof for civil commitment?

Answer: Yes.

Frank Addington's mother filed a petition requesting the involuntary commitment of her son after he threatened her. He had a history of multiple prior hospitalizations. Mr. Addington requested a trial by jury to decide about his need for commitment. The judge instructed the jury to consider whether Mr. Addington was mentally ill and dangerous based on "clear and convincing evidence." At the 6-day trial, two psychiatrists who had evaluated Mr. Addington opined that he had schizophrenia and was "probably dangerous both to himself and to others." The jury found that he met criteria; he was indefinitely involuntarily committed to Austin State Hospital. Mr. Addington appealed to the Texas Court of Civil Appeals, claiming that due process required a finding "beyond a reasonable doubt" (criminal conviction). The Court of Civil Appeals agreed, but on further appeal, the Texas Supreme Court reversed and said that, in keeping with precedent, the burden of proof for civil commitment is "preponderance of the evidence." The U.S. Supreme Court granted certiorari given the obvious confusion about this issue. In a unanimous decision, it found that an intermediate burden of proof by "clear and convincing evidence" was the most appropriate balance of individual rights and state's interests. It wrote, "One who is suffering from a debilitating mental illness and in need of treatment is neither wholly at liberty nor free of stigma."

PARHAM V. J.R., 442 U.S. 584 (1979)

Link to case: http://caselaw.lp.findlaw.com/scripts/getcase.pl?navby=case&court=us&vol=442&page=584

Question: Is an adversarial hearing required for the hospitalization of a minor whose parents or guardian has requested such action?

Answer: No.

This case represented a class action in which J.R., a minor, was an appellee. He was removed from his parents' care at 3 months of age and was subsequently placed in seven successive foster homes. At age 7, J.R.'s seventh set of foster parents successfully applied for his admission to Central State Hospital in Georgia. Voluntary admission criteria per Georgia statute included the requirements of mental illness and suitability for hospital treatment, along with a requirement to discharge any child who has "sufficiently recovered" or improved such that hospitalization is no longer "desirable." Clinicians periodically reviewed J.R.'s need for hospitalization, and attempts were made to find placement for him in foster homes. He filed suit, along with others, requesting that he be transferred to a less restrictive setting. The district court agreed, finding that the mechanism for voluntary hospitalization of minors violated constitutional due process in light of the significant deprivation of liberty entailed in hospitalization. It found a "right after notice to be heard before an impartial tribunal" to be essential and that psychiatry was too "inexact" and sources of information potentially too unreliable to protect the liberty interests of children. It ordered that Georgia release at least 46 children into specialized community treatment. The U.S. Supreme Court heard the case and reversed the district court decision. It reasoned that in light of the medical questions raised in an application for voluntary admission, "due process is not violated by use of informal, traditional medical investigative techniques." It also noted the risks of intrusion into the parent-child relationship and the potential impact on the long-term treatment of the child with the introduction of an adversarial hearing. It did not find a compelling difference between requests for admission from natural parents of a child as compared with requests from state guardians (as in J.R.'s case).

CHAPTER 7

Right to Die

ELIZABETH FORD

CRUZAN V. DIRECTOR OF MISSOURI DEPARTMENT OF MENTAL HEALTH, 497 U.S. 261 (1990)

Link to case: http://caselaw.lp.findlaw.com/scripts/getcase.pl?navby=case&court=us&vol=497&page=261

Question: Is it constitutionally acceptable for a state to require the burden of proof for removal of life-sustaining treatment from an incompetent individual to be clear and convincing evidence?

Answer: Yes.

Nancy Cruzan was in a motor vehicle accident in 1983 that resulted in severe anoxic brain injury and eventual decline into a persistent vegetative state that required artificial nutrition and hydration. Once it was clear that she would not recover, her parents asked the Missouri hospital where she was residing to terminate the artificial nutrition. Ms. Cruzan did not have any advance directives. By this time, Ms. Cruzan had been in a vegetative state for years. The hospital insisted on a court order for treatment termination; the state trial court granted that order, claiming a constitutional right to avoid "death-prolonging procedures" and in light of a prior conversation Ms. Cruzan had had with a friend about quality-of-life issues. Before the artificial feedings were discontinued, however, the Supreme Court of Missouri reversed the trial court based in part on findings that the evidence presented did not meet the "clear and convincing" standard required in Missouri and that Ms. Cruzan's parents could not automatically become her decision-makers without required legal procedure. The U.S. Supreme Court heard the case and found, in a 5–4 decision, that this standard was appropriate given the competing interests of Ms. Cruzan's liberty and the state's legitimate interest in preserving life. Following this decision, Ms. Cruzan's parents eventually produced further evidence of her wishes, and the Missouri court granted the removal of the feeding tube.

WASHINGTON V. GLUCKSBERG, 521 U.S. 702 (1997)

Link to case: http://scholar.google.com/scholar_case?case=17920279791882194984

Question: Does the ban on physician-assisted suicide of competent terminally ill adults in the state of Washington violate the Due Process Clause of the Fourteenth Amendment?

Answer: No.

Harold Glucksberg and three other physicians, along with three terminally ill patients and a nonprofit organization offering counseling to patients considering physician-assisted suicide, sued the State of Washington and claimed that Washington's ban on physician-assisted suicide was unconstitutional by violating Fourteenth Amendment liberty interests in making end-of-life decisions. The district court agreed and also found that the Washington law violated the Equal Protection Clause. A panel of judges from the U.S. Court of Appeals for the Ninth Circuit reversed and stated that there was no precedent for allowing someone to kill him- or herself. The entire appellate court then reheard the case and changed its decision, finding that the Constitution elucidated a "right to die." The U.S. Supreme Court reversed the Ninth Circuit, reasoning that there is no tradition of a right to die in the United States; that Washington State has a legitimate interest in preserving life, protecting vulnerable patients, and preserving the medical profession; and that a right to die is not a fundamental liberty interest. The Court issued the opinions for this case and *Vacco v. Quill* on the same day, striking down both elements of the Fourteenth Amendment claims (substantive due process and equal protection).

VACCO V. QUILL, 521 U.S. 793 (1997)

Link to case: http://scholar.google.com/scholar_case?case=10644975876581235704

Question: Does an individual have a right to physician-assisted suicide under the Equal Protection Clause of the Fourteenth Amendment?

Answer: No.

Timothy Quill, Samuel Klagsbrun, and Howard Grossman were three physicians in New York who filed a suit, along with three terminally ill patients, against the state's attorney general, Dennis Vacco. The physicians reported that the New York State ban on physician-assisted suicide made it illegal for them to practice consistent with their standards by prescribing lethal doses of medication for their "mentally competent, terminally ill" patients. The physicians and patients argued an equal protection claim that competent patients were allowed to refuse life-sustaining treatment yet were not allowed to seek the assistance of a physician to end their life. The district court dismissed the case, finding a significant difference between intentional action to end life and a natural end to life. However, the U.S. Court of Appeals for the Second Circuit reversed and found Dr. Quill's and others' arguments compelling. The U.S. Supreme Court heard the case and in a unanimous decision found in favor of New York State. It wrote that mentally competent people were entitled to refuse life-sustaining treatment, but that "no one is permitted to assist a suicide." It did not find the two situations to be similar classes of individuals entitled to equal protection.

CHAPTER 8

Right to Treatment

BIPIN SUBEDI

ROUSE V. CAMERON, 373 F.2D 451 (1966)

Link to case: http://scholar.google.com/scholar_case?case=10042825042511534924

Question: Do hospitalized insanity acquittees have a right to treatment?

Answer: Yes.

Charles Rouse was arrested in Washington, DC, carrying a 45-caliber revolver and 600 rounds of ammunition. He successfully pled insanity on a misdemeanor weapons violation, a charge that carried a maximum sentence of 1 year, and was sent to St. Elizabeth's Hospital. While at St. Elizabeth's, Mr. Rouse was only intermittently engaged in group/individual therapy and was not prescribed medication. After 3 years of hospitalization, he petitioned Dale Cameron, the superintendent, for release on the grounds that there was no basis for continued hospitalization if he was not receiving treatment. The DC District Court denied a hearing, stating that its jurisdiction was limited to determinations of sanity, not right to treatment. The DC Court of Appeals agreed to hear the case and ruled that a district code citing a statutory right to treatment for civilly committed patients applied to insanity acquittees. In the ruling, Judge David Bazelon stated that dangerousness determinations should be based on symptoms of mental illness and not on the crime itself. He defined treatment broadly as an "effort" to improve health and alluded to Rouse's right to treatment under the Due Process Clause of the Fourteenth Amendment. The case was reversed and remanded with instructions for the lower court to evaluate the need for hospitalization based on mental illness criteria.

WYATT V. STICKNEY, 344 F. SUPP. 373 (1972)

Link to case: http://scholar.google.com/scholar_case?case=15111627758791375629

Question: Are individuals civilly committed for mental illness or mental retardation entitled, by the U.S. Constitution, to minimally adequate standards for psychiatric treatment?

Answer: Yes.

Ricky Wyatt, a patient at Bryce Hospital in Tuscaloosa, Alabama, sued the hospital over poor conditions and treatment on behalf of other patients confined at Bryce and several employees. At the time, Alabama ranked 50th in the United States in per-patient expenditures per day. In addition, state losses following a change in tobacco taxation led to the termination of 99 employees months prior to the initiation of the suit. The District Court in Alabama agreed that treatment was grossly deficient and gave the defendants 6 months to improve conditions; 6 months later, the court determined that the defendants had failed to do so. It ruled that confining an individual for therapeutic purposes while not providing adequate treatment was a violation of substantive due process under the Fourteenth Amendment. The court subsequently held formal hearings with mental health professionals to determine the minimal constitutional standards for the treatment of psychiatric inpatients. It determined that this included (1) a humane psychological and physical environment; (2) qualified staff in numbers sufficient to administer adequate treatment; and (3) individualized treatment plans. Requirements for staffing included two psychiatrists and 12 nurses per 250 patients. The same court extended this ruling to institutions caring for the mentally disabled shortly after.

YOUNGBERG V. ROMEO, 457 U.S. 307 (1982)

Link to case: http://scholar.google.com/scholar_case?case=7713558129166322035

Question: Does the Fourteenth Amendment right to liberty include freedom from bodily restraint, safe conditions, and minimally adequate skills to reduce the need for restraint for intellectually disabled individuals who are civilly committed?

Answer: Yes.

Nicholas Romeo was a 33-year-old man with a mental capacity of an 18-month-old and an IQ score between 8 and 10. He had a history of violence and was committed to Pennhurst State School and Hospital in Pennsylvania after his father's death. At Pennhurst, Mr. Romeo suffered from multiple injuries on at least 63 occasions over 3 years. Mr. Romeo's mother filed suit against Mr. Youngberg, the superintendent at Pennhurst, claiming Eighth Amendment constitutional violations that Mr. Romeo was receiving inadequate care and had a right to safe conditions, freedom from bodily restraint, and minimally adequate skills development ("habilitation") to reduce the need for restraint. The jury found for Mr. Romeo, but the Court of Appeals for the Third Circuit reversed and remanded for a new trial, ruling that the Fourteenth Amendment's protection of liberty interests should be the guiding principle in the decision. The U.S. Supreme Court agreed to hear the case and ruled that institutionalized persons are dependent on the state and therefore have a significant liberty interest that implicates due process protections, including the rights stated in Mr. Romeo's original claim. It also reasoned that, in light of the potential for legitimate need for restraint to protect safety, professional judgment—an assessment of whether an action substantially deviated from the standard of care—was an appropriate measure of whether the above-mentioned rights had been violated.

CHAPTER 9

Right to Refuse Treatment

REBECCA LEWIS

APPLICATION OF THE PRESIDENT AND DIRECTORS OF GEORGETOWN UNIVERSITY, 331 F.2D 1000 (1964)

Link to case: http://law.justia.com/cases/federal/appellate-courts/F2/331/1010/445992/

Question: Does imminent danger of death trump an incompetent patient's religious objections to emergency medical treatment in the District of Columbia?

Answer: Yes.

Jesse Jones was a patient at Georgetown University Hospital in Washington, DC. Her husband brought her to the hospital for emergency care after she lost two-thirds of her blood from a ruptured ulcer. Blood transfusions were necessary to save her life, but Mrs. Jones and her husband refused to consent to the blood transfusions based on their religious beliefs as Jehovah's Witnesses. When death without transfusion became imminent, the hospital applied to the district court for permission to administer blood transfusions. The district court denied the application. The hospital then applied to Judge Wright as a member of the DC Circuit Court of Appeals for an emergency writ. Judge Wright confirmed the medical facts with the doctors. He spoke with Mrs. Jones's husband, who said that on religious grounds he would not approve a blood transfusion, but that if the court ordered the transfusion, the responsibility was not his. Judge Wright then tried to communicate with Mrs. Jones; her only audible reply was "against my will." Judge Wright found her incompetent to make medical decisions in her compromised state of health. He granted permission for blood transfusions "to save her life" and stated that death could have made the case moot.

SUPERINTENDENT OF BELCHERTOWN STATE SCHOOL ET AL. V. JOSEPH SAIKEWICZ, 370 N.E.2D 417 (1977)

Link to case: http://scholar.google.com/scholar_case?case=2165107287898894579

Question: Is substituted judgment an appropriate decision-making standard for a legally appointed guardian to employ when making medical decisions for his or her ward?

Answer: Yes.

Joseph Saikewicz, a resident of the Belchertown State School in Massachusetts, was 67 years old and had an IQ of 10. He was diagnosed with leukemia and was incapable of giving consent for treatment. The superintendent petitioned for appointment of a guardian ad litem to make treatment decisions. The guardian ad litem recommended that treatment for Mr. Saikewicz would not be in his best interests based on the following assessment: (1) the treatment (chemotherapy) would cause significant adverse effects that Mr. Saikewicz would not understand, (2) there was a low chance of remission, and (3) there would be only a limited extension of life if remission occurred. The probate court agreed with the substituted judgment of the guardian and ordered that no treatment be administered. Although Mr. Saikewicz died in the interim, the probate court requested review of this decision by the Supreme Court of Massachusetts. That court concluded that substituted judgment for incompetent patients was the appropriate decision-making standard and that "to presume that the incompetent person must always be subjected to what many rational and intelligent persons may decline is to downgrade the status of the incompetent person by placing a lesser value on his intrinsic human worth and vitality."

IN THE MATTER OF THE GUARDIANSHIP OF RICHARD ROE, III, 383 MASS. 415 (1981)

Link to case: http://masscases.com/cases/sjc/383/383mass415.html#back23

Question: Can a legally appointed guardian of an individual in Massachusetts with mental illness consent to involuntary, nonemergent administration of antipsychotic medication for that individual?

Answer: No.

Richard Roe III was diagnosed with paranoid schizophrenia as a teenager and was eventually hospitalized at Northampton State Hospital, where he refused antipsychotic medications. His father was appointed as guardian after his discharge from the hospital. The probate court ordered that Mr. Roe's father would have the authority to consent to forcible administration of medication. The guardian ad litem, appointed to represent Mr. Roe in the probate hearing, appealed. The Massachusetts Supreme Court held that the appointment of a guardian was warranted and that the evidence was appropriately tested under a "preponderance of the evidence" standard of proof. However, the court ruled that it was an error to empower the guardian (Mr. Roe's father) to consent for forcible administration of medications. The court concluded that, absent an emergency, in a noninstitutionalized patient, antipsychotic medications may be administered forcibly only when ordered by a judge using a substituted judgment standard. It determined that if the ward, if competent, would accept the medications, the judge should order administration. If determined that the substituted judgment would be to refuse treatment, then the judge should consider whether there is a state interest sufficient to override the decision to refuse (e.g., interest in preventing violence). If the judge finds that there is such a state interest, then an extended substituted judgment determination must be used to choose between options for satisfying this interest (e.g., involuntary commitment vs. forced medication).

RENNIE V. KLEIN, 720 F.2D 266 (1983)

Link to case: http://scholar.google.com/scholar_case?case=11241063757300199813

Question: In New Jersey, do individuals civilly committed for psychiatric treatment have a right to refuse antipsychotic medication?

Answer: Yes.

During his 12th hospitalization at a New Jersey state hospital, John Rennie initiated a suit claiming a constitutional right of involuntarily hospitalized mentally ill patients to refuse antipsychotic medications. The district court agreed. The U.S. Court of Appeals for the Third Circuit found that the constitutional right to refuse treatment existed, but it found that the administrative procedures outlined in New Jersey's Administrative Bulletin (which required a hospital administrative review prior to forcible administration of medications) provided adequate protection and satisfied due process. The court added that the medication administered must be the least restrictive treatment available. This decision was then appealed to the U.S. Supreme Court. The Court instructed the Third Circuit to reconsider the case in view of the Supreme Court's finding in *Youngberg v Romeo*, which adopted a standard of "professional judgment" instead of the "least restrictive means." The New Jersey procedures require that the physician explain reasons for medication, the benefits and risks of medication, and alternative courses of action. Additionally, the proposed treatment must be reviewed and approved by other professional staff. Upon reconsideration, the Third Circuit found that the New Jersey regulations satisfied the professional judgment standard. This case represents a treatment-driven approach to establishing a patient's right to refuse treatment.

ROGERS V. COMMISSIONER, 458 N.E.2D 308 (1983)

Link to case: http://freedom-center.org/pdf/rogersruling.pdf

Question: In Massachusetts, can an involuntarily committed patient refuse psychiatric medication?

Answer: Yes.

Rubie Rogers was one of the plaintiffs in a class action against the commissioner of the Department of Mental Health in Massachusetts that challenged the practice of medicating patients against their will. The district court found that forcibly medicating hospitalized patients in nonemergency situations was prohibited, but it denied damages. Both parties appealed. The U.S. Court of Appeals for the First Circuit affirmed the denial of damages and also affirmed that mentally ill patients have a constitutionally protected right to refuse treatment. However, the court of appeals expanded the meaning of emergency to balance police power interest and to consider if a patient's heath would significantly deteriorate without medications. The U.S. Supreme Court granted certiorari, vacated the judgment, and remanded the case to the court of appeals to specify how the patient's rights were protected. The court of appeals then sent the case back to the district court and requested responses to multiple questions regarding involuntary medication. The district court specified the following: 1) competency and substituted judgment determinations must be made in court by a judge; 2) a substituted judgment treatment decision must be made before a hospitalized patient can be forcibly medicated; and 3) emergencies (e.g., preventing violence or preventing the immediate and irreversible deterioration of serious mental illness) are exceptions to these requirements. Even though this case was ultimately decided by the district court, it did so under the guidance of the U.S. Supreme Court. This case is an example of a rights-driven approach to a patient's right to refuse treatment (in contrast to *Rennie v. Klein*—a treatment-driven approach).

CHAPTER 10

Questions on Institutional Treatment Guidelines

QUESTIONS

1. What does the principle of "least restrictive alternative" mean?
   A. Keeping someone in jail or prison no longer than his or her sentence
   B. Using restraints for only 2 hours at a time on psychiatric units
   C. Using only a level of force, coercion, or restriction needed to ensure safety
   D. Using justice as a means of enforcing the law

2. In order to remove life-sustaining treatment from an incompetent individual without existing advance directives, the required burden of proof is:
   A. Preponderance of the evidence
   B. Clear and convincing evidence
   C. Beyond a reasonable doubt
   D. With reasonable medical certainty

3. What is substituted judgment?
   A. When a guardian or judge determines the choice a currently incompetent individual would make if he or she were competent
   B. When a doctor is asked to determine the most medically appropriate treatment for an incompetent individual
   C. When a judge is asked to determine what treatment choice the majority of people in the same medical position as the incompetent individual would make
   D. When an incompetent individual's next of kin makes the decision about treatment for that individual

4. What U.S. Supreme Court case most defined the dangerousness standard for civil commitment?
   A. *Lessard v. Schmidt*
   B. *Lake v. Cameron*
   C. *O'Connor v. Donaldson*
   D. *Addington v. Texas*

5. Which court gave the final ruling in *Youngberg v. Romeo*?
   A. U.S. District Court
   B. U.S. Court of Appeals
   C. U.S. Supreme Court
   D. Family court

6. Is physician-assisted suicide allowable under the American Medical Association (AMA) guidelines?
   A. Yes.
   B. No.
   C. The AMA does not comment on physician-assisted suicide.
   D. The AMA allows physician-assisted suicide in certain circumstances.

7. In *Rouse v. Cameron*, the Washington, DC, statutory right to treatment that applied to civilly committed patients was found to also apply to which other class of individuals?
   A. Individuals with developmental disabilities
   B. Insanity acquittees
   C. Prisoners
   D. Pretrial detainees

8. Can medical professionals provide emergency lifesaving medical treatment to an incompetent person against his or her will?
   A. Yes. Physicians are always permitted to treat incompetent individuals, as long as it is the appropriate medical treatment, even in a nonemergency situation.
   B. Yes. If the medical treatment is lifesaving and there is imminent risk of death, physicians can provide the treatment.
   C. Yes, but only if there is a judicial court order for treatment.
   D. No. Medical professionals are never permitted to treat individuals against their will, even if the individual is incompetent.

9. In *Wyatt v. Stickney*, the U.S. District Court ruled that the minimal constitutional requirements for the treatment of committed patients were:
   A. Humane psychological and physical environment, qualified staff in numbers sufficient to administer adequate treatment, right to legal representation

QUESTIONS ON INSTITUTIONAL TREATMENT GUIDELINES (61)

B. Humane psychological and physical environment, qualified staff in numbers sufficient to administer adequate treatment, and adequate funding
C. Qualified staff in numbers sufficient to administer adequate treatment, individualized treatment plans, and adequate funding
D. Humane psychological and physical environment, qualified staff in numbers sufficient to administer adequate treatment, and individualized treatment plans

10. The U.S. Supreme Court has found which of the following to be a compelling argument against physician-assisted suicide?
    A. The difference between letting a patient die and making a patient die.
    B. Competent individuals should have a right to choose their manner of death.
    C. Competent people can refuse lifesaving treatments.
    D. All of the above.

11. The legal burden of proof for civil commitment in the United States is:
    A. Beyond reasonable doubt
    B. Reasonable medical certainty
    C. Preponderance of the evidence
    D. Clear and convincing evidence
    E. Without due cause

12. In the Matter of Richard Roe, III was a case involving an outpatient minor. Based on that case, does a guardian have the authority to consent to forcible medication of his or her ward?
    A. No. Medications cannot be administered against someone's will if the person is not hospitalized.
    B. No. Only a court can determine if forcible medication can be ordered for an outpatient.
    C. Yes. The courts appoint a guardian, and this guardian then has the authority to consent for medically appropriate treatment, even if it is against the ward's wishes.
    D. Yes. A review between the guardian and the ward's physician is appropriate.

13. In what circumstance does an individual have a right to an adversarial hearing?
    A. If a minor, when one's parents apply for voluntary admission
    B. All voluntary admissions, regardless of age of the individual

C. When facing involuntary hospitalization
D. When a request for release from a medical unit is denied

14. According to the U.S. Supreme Court, physician-assisted suicide:
    A. Is constitutional under the Fourteenth Amendment
    B. Reasonably allows an individual to exercise his or her autonomy
    C. Should not be an issue decided at the Supreme Court level
    D. Is not rationally related to legitimate government interests
    E. Is akin to allowing a patient to die of natural causes

15. Of the following choices, which legal or ethical principles are most at odds in civil commitment?
    A. Nonmaleficence versus police power
    B. Beneficence versus autonomy
    C. Autonomy versus police power
    D. Autonomy versus nonmaleficence
    E. Justice versus beneficence

16. According to *Washington v. Glucksberg* and *Vacco v. Quill*, state bans on physician-assisted suicide do not violate:
    A. The Eighth Amendment
    B. The First Amendment
    C. The Fourteenth Amendment
    D. The Sixth Amendment
    E. The Second Amendment

17. In *Rennie v. Klein*, a treatment-driven model of adjudicating cases involving treatment refusal was found to be sound. What reasoning was used?
    A. The courts should decide these cases based on substituted judgment.
    B. Professional judgment should guide treatment refusal decisions.
    C. The judicial system should tightly monitor all clinical decisions regarding treatment refusal.
    D. Specific treatment should be implemented once an order to medicate someone against his or her will is obtained.

18. Protections for patients involuntarily committed to a psychiatric hospital include:
    A. Right to legal representation
    B. Right to leave the hospital against medical advice
    C. Right to a choose their doctor
    D. Right to choose the hospital to which they are committed

19. A hospitalized patient of yours is in a persistent vegetative state following a major car accident and is receiving artificial nutrition and hydration to stay alive. He does not have any written advance directives, but his older brother wishes to remove the feeding tube and allow his brother's life to take a natural course, even if that ends in death. What would be the best first step?
    A. Tell the brother that the tube cannot ever be removed.
    B. Consult the hospital risk management department.
    C. Talk to other family members about their wishes.
    D. Remove the feeding tube.

20. Does an incompetent individual have the right to refuse life-prolonging medical treatment?
    A. Yes, but only if that individual had made his or her desire to avoid such treatment known prior to becoming incompetent.
    B. Yes, but only if it is shown that the majority of people in a similar situation would refuse such treatment.
    C. No. If treatment can prolong life, and the individual is incompetent, he or she cannot refuse such treatment.
    D. Yes. Even if the individual has never been competent, a legally appointed guardian can make the decision.

21. Which of the following statements best describes the procedure for civilly committing an individual being released from prison?
    A. The individual must be assessed by at least three psychiatrists, all board certified by the ABPN.
    B. The individual should be afforded the right to a jury trial the same as for nonprisoners being civilly committed.
    C. The individual should be released from prison into the community before being assessed for civil commitment.
    D. The individual should be found in need of civil commitment beyond a reasonable doubt.

22. The U.S. Supreme Court defined what standard for determining Fourteen Amendment violations of due process for civilly committed, intellectually disabled individuals?
    A. Substantial necessity
    B. Professional judgment
    C. Compelling necessity
    D. Reasonable medical certainty
    E. Preponderance of the evidence

ANSWERS

1. **C**

    "Least restrictive alternative" is a concept that describes respecting an individual's autonomy and liberty as much as safety permits. It is mentioned frequently in legal cases involving civil commitment and patient rights. Answers (A) and (B) are examples of practices that conform to the "least restrictive alternative" principle. Answer (D) relates to issues of therapeutic jurisprudence and police power, neither of which is directly related to least restrictive alternative.

2. **B**

    The issue was decided in the U.S. Supreme Court case *Cruzan v. Director of Missouri Department of Mental Health* in 1990. It involved a woman in a persistent vegetative state who did not have advance directives and whose parents wished to withdraw life-sustaining nutrition and hydration. The Court reasoned that the state had a strong interest in preserving life and that the "clear and convincing" standard appropriately weighted that interest against an individual's liberty interest. Answers (A) and (C) are lower and higher standards of proof, respectively. Answer (D) is the level of certainty physicians use in offering expert opinions.

3. **A**

    Substituted judgment is used to determine what an incompetent individual would choose if he or she were competent. In *In the Matter of the Guardianship of Richard Roe, III*, the Massachusetts Supreme Court outlined the important factors to consider when determining substituted judgment: (1) the ward's expressed preferences, (2) the ward's religious beliefs, (3) the impact upon the ward's family, (4) the probability of adverse side effects of treatment, (5) the consequences if treatment is refused, and (6) the prognosis with treatment.

4. **C**

    O'Connor v. Donaldson was a U.S. Supreme Court case that highlighted dangerousness, along with mental illness, as the required criteria for civil commitment. *Lessard v. Schmidt* (Wisconsin) and *Lake v. Cameron* (Washington, DC) were not U.S. Supreme Court cases. *Addington v. Texas* defined the burden of proof for involuntary psychiatric hospitalization but did not define the clinical requirements.

QUESTIONS ON INSTITUTIONAL TREATMENT GUIDELINES (65)

5. **C**

   Youngberg v. Romeo was the first U.S. Supreme Court decision to address the issue of right to treatment. The Alabama District Court ruled in *Wyatt v. Stickney*, and the DC Court of Appeals ruled in *Rouse v. Cameron*. Family courts do not have the jurisdiction to address constitutional matters.

6. **B**

   The AMA comments on physician-assisted suicide in Opinion 2.211 (http://www.ama-assn.org//ama/pub/physician-resources/medical-ethics/code-medical-ethics/opinion2211.page). In it, the AMA finds that the practice is "incompatible with the physician's role as healer." It does not list any exceptions to this position.

7. **B**

   Charles Rouse was an insanity acquittee and petitioned for release, stating that he was not receiving treatment where he had been hospitalized following his acquittal. Although a district court statute clearly outlined a right to treatment for civilly committed patients, it was unclear, prior to this case, if this applied to those who were found not criminally responsible secondary to mental illness. In *Rouse v. Cameron*, the DC Circuit Court of Appeals ruled that once found not responsible, Mr. Rouse was effectively a civil patient and therefore had the same right to treatment. The case does not discuss incarcerated individuals or individuals with developmental disabilities.

8. **B**

   In *Application of the President and Directors of Georgetown University*, a patient was at imminent risk of death from a bleeding ulcer and was refusing blood transfusions. A judge determined that the patient was incompetent and that treatment should be provided to save her life. He noted that waiting for a court hearing would have mooted the issue because the patient would die before a hearing. Physicians are not permitted to treat incompetent patients against their will in non-emergency settings. Instead, they must consult a legal surrogate (e.g., power of attorney, court-appointed guardian).

9. **D**

   In *Wyatt v. Stickney*, the court ruled that patients had the rights outlined in (D) and provided specific guidelines in the appendix of the ruling. Lack of funding was not considered to be a valid excuse in failing to provide the necessary services.

10. **A**

In their decisions in *Washington v. Glucksberg* and *Vacco v. Quill*, the U.S. Supreme Court emphasized the difference between allowing a patient to die naturally (e.g., not initiating extraordinary measures) and causing a patient die (physician-assisted suicide). Answers (B) and (C) are arguments in favor of physician-assisted suicide but were not compelling enough to the Court.

11. **D**

Since *Addington v. Texas*, the minimum burden of proof for the fact-finder (e.g., judge or jury) in a civil commitment proceeding is "clear and convincing evidence." The U.S. Supreme Court considered the standard of "beyond reasonable doubt" (used in criminal matters) so high that it would limit access to hospitalization for mentally ill patients because few would reach that burden of proof. "Preponderance of the evidence" (more likely than not) was considered so low that the autonomy rights of individuals with mental illness would not be protected, and unfair hospitalizations would occur. "Clear and convincing evidence" was considered a reasonable compromise. "Reasonable medical certainty" is the standard that an evaluating clinician must use in determining whether or not to initiate civil commitment. It is equivalent to "more likely than not." "Without due cause" is not a recognized standard.

12. **B**

In *In the Matter of the Guardianship of Richard Roe, III*, the father of Richard Roe was appointed his guardian after his discharge from a state hospital and authorized to consent to forcible administration of medications for Richard Roe. This was appealed, and the Massachusetts Supreme Court found that in a noninstitutionalized patient, absent an emergency, medications could be administered forcibly only when ordered by a judge.

13. **C**

Individuals facing involuntary hospitalization have a right to an adversarial hearing, among other due process rights (see *Lessard v. Schmidt*). The case of *Parham v. J.R.* found that Georgia's practice of voluntary admission for minors was constitutional and did not require an adversarial hearing. Although Parham was a case about a class action related to minors, adults who request voluntary admission do not have a right to an adversarial hearing. Individuals who are admitted to a medical unit and are denied release upon request can, if competent and not

QUESTIONS ON INSTITUTIONAL TREATMENT GUIDELINES (67)

in an emergency situation, sign out against medical advice without a hearing.

14. **D**

    The U.S. Supreme Court heard two major state cases about physician-assisted suicide in 1997: *Washington v. Glucksberg* (Washington) and *Vacco v. Quill* (New York). In each, the Court found that the state could ban the procedure according to the Fourteenth Amendment. It was not swayed by arguments about an individual's right to die (autonomy). The Court found a significant difference between letting a patient die by natural causes and hastening his or her death (likened to killing a patient). Prominent arguments in each case were the respective state's reasonable and legitimate interests in preserving life and protecting vulnerable populations.

15. **C**

    All of the ethical principles described are frequently considered in psychiatric practice; however, autonomy and police power are the most in conflict during civil commitment decisions. Autonomy means the ability to be one's own person and to act in one's own interests, regardless of the input from others. Police power is a right of the government, conferred by the Tenth Amendment of the U.S. Constitution, to make policies that protect the safety and welfare of the community. In civil commitment decisions, a mentally ill individual's autonomy to make treatment decisions is balanced against the state's right to restrict the liberty of those who may be dangerous to society. Nonmaleficence is the concept in the Hippocratic oath commonly known as "first, do no harm." It, along with beneficence (do what is in the best interests of the patient), is a common principle in clinical practice. Justice is the fair treatment of all individuals in a society.

16. **C**

    Both cases were Fourteenth Amendment claims, but each emphasized a different part of the amendment. *Washington v. Glucksberg* was an equal protection claim, and *Vacco v. Quill* was a due process claim. The Eighth and Sixth Amendments are both related to criminal justice, the First Amendment has to do with freedom of speech and religion, and the Second Amendment has to do with a right to bear arms.

17. **B**

    Rennie v. Klein exemplifies the treatment-driven model. In this case, it was found that a constitutional right to refuse treatment existed, but that the administrative procedures outlined in New Jersey's

Administrative Bulletin (which required a hospital administrative review prior to forcible administration of medications) provided adequate protection of patients' rights and found that the decision to medicate a patient against his or her wishes must be the result of professional judgment (to protect the patient from inappropriate or unnecessary medication). *Rogers v. Commissioner* exemplifies the rights-driven model. In this case, the courts found that patients are entitled to a judicial hearing, and that the court determines competency and then makes a determination about treatment over objection based on a substituted judgment standard.

18. **A**

    Involuntary civil commitment is considered a significant deprivation of liberty in the United States. As a result, patients who are involuntarily committed are entitled to contest that deprivation through legal means, such as legal representation—provided free of charge for those who cannot afford an attorney—and a court hearing. Involuntarily committed psychiatric patients do not have a specific right to leave against medical advice, to choose their own doctor, or to choose the hospital to which they are committed. Patients hospitalized for other reasons (e.g., medical/surgical) are able to leave against medical advice assuming that they have the capacity to make such a decision.

19. **B**

    Although the patient's brother may be successful in having the feeding tube removed if he can present clear and convincing evidence of his brother's wish not to receive life-sustaining treatment (*Cruzan v. Director of Missouri Department of Mental Health*), family members cannot automatically make end-of-life decisions for incompetent relatives. It may be advisable to speak with multiple family members when, as a physician, you are considering a difficult clinical decision, but in this case, it is advisable to first consult the hospital risk management department to identify your legal and ethical responsibilities in the state in which you practice.

20. **D**

    In *Superintendent of Belchertown State School et al. v. Joseph Saikewicz*, Mr. Saikewicz was an individual with an IQ of 10. It was difficult to determine substituted judgment for him, as he had never been competent. His guardian recommended against treatment with chemotherapy for leukemia, given Saikewicz's inability to comprehend the treatment or the reason for the many adverse side effects, and given the only limited extension of life as a possible benefit of treatment. The court agreed with this recommendation and asked for review from the Massachusetts Supreme Court. It was concluded that the guardian's recommendation against treatment was appropriate, as the incompetent person should not simply be subjected to what most competent people would decide.

21. **B**

    Baxstrom v. Herold was a U.S. Supreme Court decision stating that mentally ill prisoners nearing release from custody should be afforded the same procedural due process rights for civil commitment as civilians. The Court did not find a substantial difference in the populations to justify a different standard. The case did not directly involve the specific requirements of the certifying psychiatrists, much less that they be board certified. There was no mention that the individual should be released to the community first; this would likely be too much of a public safety risk to be acceptable. Although *Addington v. Texas* (1990) had not yet been decided (establishing a burden of proof for civil commitment), this case did not address the burden of proof issue.

22. **B**

    Youngberg v. Romeo was a U.S. Supreme Court case that addressed the due process rights of intellectually disabled, involuntarily committed individuals, including a right to freedom from restraint and safety of confinement. There was disagreement at the circuit court level about what standard should be used in determining violations, since in some instances restraints are necessary. The circuit court suggested "substantial necessity" and "compelling necessity"; however, the Supreme Court determined that it was "professional judgment."

SECTION III

Child and Adolescent Issues

The cases included in this section address issues affecting vulnerable youths and are related to the general practice of child psychiatry, which includes the areas of child abuse, child custody, juvenile justice, education rights, and individuals with disabilities. Issues such as mandated reporting to protect vulnerable individuals are now nearly universal concepts for practicing physicians and other allied health professionals and also extend to law enforcement and educators. The "best interests of the child" standard is the bedrock of decisions in child custody matters and also extends to various legal approaches to placement decisions for children involved in the child welfare system.

In re Gault is a landmark case in juvenile justice and was critical in extending due process protections for juvenile offenders. This case has been foundational in the evolution of how young offenders are processed through the juvenile delinquency system and reflected the need for establishing greater protections and civil rights. Inasmuch as the more lax due process standards prior to *Gault* were justified by the treatment orientation of the juvenile justice system, the changes resulting from *Gault* (and justification for same) became the benchmarks for later consideration of the rights of individuals with mental illness in ostensibly treatment-focused civil commitment proceedings.

The Education for All Handicapped Children Act also reflected the need to buttress constitutional protections for another vulnerable group of children, those with intellectual and developmental disorders (disabilities). The EAHCA case required all federally funded public schools to provide equal access to education in addition to one free meal a day for children with intellectual and developmental disabilities, citing the Fourteenth Amendment equal protection under the law.

CHAPTER 11

Child Abuse Reporting

SHAWN S. SIDHU AND ERAKA BATH

LANDEROS V. FLOOD, 551 P.2D 389 (1976)

Link to case: http://scholar.google.com/scholar_case?case=3441539196251667835

Question: Can a physician who fails to diagnose battered child syndrome be found liable for subsequent injuries to the child?

Answer: Yes.

Gita Landeros, an 11-month-old baby, was taken by her mother to a local hospital for evaluation. A diagnostic workup by Dr. A. J. Flood revealed multiple bruises on baby Landeros's back and a leg fracture most commonly resulting from significant twisting force. She was treated and discharged back to the care of her mother. Shortly thereafter, baby Landeros presented again to another hospital where she was evaluated for multiple injuries, including an incompletely healed skull fracture and a left hand wound potentially severe enough to warrant amputation. She was diagnosed with battered child syndrome, and her mother and father were convicted of child abuse. The state-appointed guardian then filed a lawsuit against Dr. Flood for failure to identify physical injury secondary to maltreatment. The trial court dismissed the case, but on appeal, the Supreme Court of California ruled that the vast majority of physicians would have correctly diagnosed battered child syndrome and found in favor of baby Landeros.

The court argued that the failure to correctly diagnose the patient and alert the proper authorities ultimately resulted in increased harm to the child. Dr. Flood was ultimately held accountable for baby Landeros's subsequent injuries.

PEOPLE V. STRITZINGER, 668 P.2D 738 (1983)

Link to case: http://scholar.google.com/scholar_case?case=17744911620888675589

Question: Can a psychotherapist be compelled to report past child abuse perpetrated by a patient, without the patient's consent and without knowledge of continuing abuse?

Answer: No.

Carl Stritzinger had been sexually abusing his daughter Sarah for 15 months when Mrs. Stritzinger, his wife and Sarah's mother, learned of the molestation. Mrs. Stritzinger sought mental health services for both her husband and her daughter with Dr. Walker, a psychologist. During the course of a session, Sarah revealed that her father had sexually abused her. Pursuant to mandated reporting statutes required by California law, Dr. Walker reported the incident to child protective services. After filing his report, Dr. Walker was contacted by Deputy Buttell, in charge of investigating these allegations. During their next scheduled session, Mr. Stritzinger informed Dr. Walker of incriminating details regarding the allegations, although no new information was revealed. Deputy Buttell insisted that Dr. Walker disclose content from the therapy session and referred to part of the California Penal Code, claiming that it provided an exception to this privilege based on the abuse-reporting requirements. Invoking psychotherapist–patient privilege, Dr. Walker was hesitant to reveal content from his session and felt that he had already complied with his mandated reporting duties by contacting child protective services. He ultimately testified over objection at Mr. Stritzinger's trial, which led to a conviction. The California Supreme Court found that the trial court had erred in allowing testimony from Dr. Walker concerning the substance of the consultation with Mr. Stritzinger. The court found that Dr. Walker had been misled by Deputy Buttell; because he had already reported the incident described by Sarah and did not suspect any additional reportable activity, there was no need to violate psychotherapist–patient privilege.

DESHANEY V. WINNEBAGO, 489 U.S. 189 (1989)

Link to case: http://scholar.google.com/scholar_case?case=5543768239799414902

Question: Does a state have a constitutional obligation to protect a minor from violence perpetrated by a private citizen?

Answer: No.

Since 1 year of age, Joshua DeShaney (a minor) was repeatedly abused and victimized by his father. These incidents resulted in several emergency room visits and investigations by social workers from the Department of Social Services (DSS) in Wisconsin. At each point in the investigation, the social workers did not feel that there was significant cause to remove Joshua from his father's home, so in lieu of placing Joshua in state custody, DSS made a voluntary agreement with the father that he would enroll Joshua in preschool and that he would enroll in parenting classes. The father failed to comply with these conditions, and in March 1984, Joshua's father beat him so badly that he was in a coma and suffered permanent and severe brain damage. Joshua and his mother filed suit in district court alleging that DSS had violated the Constitution by depriving Joshua of his liberty without due process by failing to remove Joshua from his father's custody. The district court granted summary judgment for DSS; the U.S. Court of Appeals also found in favor of DSS but emphasized the difference between state and private citizen action. The U.S. Supreme Court agreed that there is no violation of the US Constitution when a governmental agency is aware that a child is being abused by a parent but fails to protect the child. The court found that the Due Process Clause refers to the state's responsibility against *state actions* and does not apply to the actions of *private* citizens. It found that the Due Process Clause of the Fourteenth Amendment does not require a state to provide protection to the general public and that the state's due process duties are not so far-reaching as to impose duties on private citizens.

CHAPTER 12

Child Custody and Parental Competencies

EILEEN P. RYAN

PAINTER V. BANNISTER, 140 N.W.2D 152 (1966)

Link to case: http://scholar.google.com/scholar_case?case=15245255595862613942

Question: Is the standard for determining child custody based on the best interests of the child?

Answer: Yes,

Harold Painter's wife died in a car accident when their son, Mark, was 5 years old. Mr. Painter requested that the maternal grandparents take temporary custody of Mark. Mr. Painter then moved to California and remarried. After 15 months, when he asked the grandparents to return Mark, they refused. Although Mr. Painter was granted custody by the trial court, the grandparents appealed to the Supreme Court of Iowa. The court awarded custody to the grandparents, noting their "stable, dependable, conventional, middle-class" environment as opposed to the father, who they noted had a "bohemian" lifestyle, had held multiple jobs, and handled money poorly. The court relied heavily on the testimony of a child psychologist who indicated that Mark's grandfather had replaced his father as the primary "father figure" in Mark's life and also emphasized the importance of stability and continuity. The psychologist was concerned that the bond between Mark and his father would not be strong enough to sustain

Mark through another wrenching loss and family transition. The court held out the legal standard for determining custody as the best interests of the child, rather than the preference of the parent.

SANTOSKY V. KRAMER, 455 U.S. 745, 102 S. CT. 1388 (1982)

Link to case: http://caselaw.lp.findlaw.com/scripts/getcase.pl?navby=case&court=us&vol=455&page=745

Question: Is preponderance of the evidence the appropriate legal burden of proof for termination of parental rights?

Answer: No.

Two siblings, Tina and John Santosky, were temporarily removed from their biological parents for neglect. A third child was immediately removed at birth. The Department of Social Services (DSS) for Ulster County in New York moved for permanent termination of the parents' rights. The Santoskys had maintained contact with their children, but the family court determined that, even with public assistance, the Santoskys were unable to care for them. Permanent termination was ruled in the children's best interests at a disposition hearing by a preponderance of the evidence, New York's standard for the termination of parental rights in neglect cases. The Santoskys challenged the standard and Kramer, the commissioner of Ulster County DSS, claiming that the burden of proof for termination should be higher. The New York Supreme Court affirmed, but the New York Court of Appeals dismissed. The U.S. Supreme Court granted certiorari and found that while the state and the parents have interests in preserving family unity, the near-equal allocation of risk between the parents and the state is unconstitutional given the relationship between parent and child. The Court ruled that the standard for terminating parental rights should be "clear and convincing evidence."

CHAPTER 13

Juvenile Rights

EILEEN P. RYAN AND ELIZABETH FORD

IN RE GAULT, 387 U.S. 1, 87 S. CT. 1428 (1967)

Link to case: http://caselaw.lp.findlaw.com/scripts/getcase.pl?navby=case&court=us&vol=387&page=1

Question: Are juvenile delinquents facing a loss of liberty entitled to similar procedural due process rights as adults charged with a crime?

Answer: Yes.

Gerald Gault was 15 years old when he and a friend were accused of making an obscene phone call to a neighbor, Mrs. Cook, allegedly commenting on her "bombers" and asking if her "cherries [were] ripe." Gerald was already on probation. He and his friend were picked up by the sheriff and brought to the Children's Detention Home in Gila County, Arizona. When Gerald's mother eventually learned of Gerald's arrest and went to the detention home, she learned that a hearing was scheduled for the next day in juvenile court. Notice about the hearing was not served on Gerald or his parents, no transcript of the hearing was made, no one was sworn in to testify, and Mrs. Cook, the complainant, was not present. At a second hearing, Mrs. Cook was again not present, despite Gerald's mother's request. A probation officer filed a report, which neither Gerald nor his parents saw, listing the charge as making lewd phone calls. Had Gerald been an adult, the maximum sentence he could have received was a $50 fine and 2 months in jail. The judge committed Gerald to a state training school until the age of 21.

Gerald's parents filed a petition for a writ of habeas corpus, which was dismissed by the Superior Court of Arizona and affirmed on appeal by the Arizona Supreme Court. The U.S. Supreme Court heard the case and determined that juveniles facing a delinquency hearing and loss of liberty are entitled to certain procedural safeguards, similar to adults charged with a crime, under the Due Process Clause of the Fourteenth Amendment. Those safeguards include written notice, a right to counsel, and the right to confront witnesses.

GRAHAM V. FLORIDA, 130 S. CT. 2011 (2010)

Link to case: http://scholar.google.com/scholar_case?case=6982366090819046045&hl=en

Question: Does the Eighth Amendment permit the sentencing of a juvenile offender to life without parole for committing a nonhomicide crime?

Answer: No.

Terrance Graham was placed on probation for a burglary and a robbery committed when he was 16 years old. Although Florida law allows discretion to prosecute 16- and 17-year-olds as adults for certain felonies, the judge in Mr. Graham's case withheld adjudication. Sometime later, now age 17, Mr. Graham was picked up for violating his probation by being involved in a robbery. Mr. Graham denied the robbery but admitted to fleeing police officers after dropping his friend at the hospital following an alleged second robbery attempt. Under Florida law, the minimum sentence he could have received for the crimes was 5 years' imprisonment; the state recommended 30 years. A presentence report recommended 4 years. The trial court found Mr. Graham guilty of the earlier charges, noting Graham's "escalating pattern of criminal conduct," and sentenced him to the maximum sentence on each charge, amounting to life imprisonment without parole, since Florida had abolished its parole system. Mr. Graham filed a motion challenging his sentence under the Eighth Amendment; it was denied. Florida's First District Court of Appeal affirmed the sentence, and the Florida Supreme Court denied review. The U.S. Supreme Court heard the case and, based on the proportionality principle (whether the punishment is proportional to the offense), concluded that the Eighth Amendment prohibits sentences of life without parole for nonhomicide defendants younger than 18, and that states must provide such defendants with "some meaningful opportunity" for release.

MILLER V. ALABAMA, 132 S. CT. 2455 (2012)

Link to case: http://scholar.google.com/scholar_case?case=6291421178853922648

Question: Does the Eighth Amendment permit mandatory sentencing of a juvenile offender to life without parole?

Answer: No.

This U.S. Supreme Court decision represents the consolidation of two cases, both involving 14-year-old defendants charged with murder. Evan Miller, with a history of multiple placements in foster care as a result of his mother's substance dependence and his stepfather's abuse, and with a history of suicide attempts beginning at the age of 6 and prior juvenile offenses, was involved in the murder of Cole Cannon following a drug deal with Evan's mother. Kuntrell Jackson was involved in a robbery of a video store that turned into a murder of the store clerk. Evan and Kuntrell were charged and then convicted as adults, since both states (Alabama and Arkansas, respectively) allowed prosecutorial discretion in moving the cases to adult court. In both cases, existing state law required a minimum sentence of life without parole for the crimes committed. Appeals courts in both states affirmed the trial court findings and sentences. The U.S. Supreme Court heard the cases and reversed the lower courts' findings, using precedents in *Roper v. Simmons* and *Graham v. Florida*, among others, as guidance. The Court found that the mandatory sentencing guidelines for murder in Alabama and Arkansas, regardless of offender age, violated the Eighth Amendment's ban on cruel and unusual punishment because adolescents are, by their developmental immaturity, less culpable and therefore less deserving of the most severe punishments. The Court did not categorically ban imposition of such a sentence but required consideration of the factors of youth in sentencing decisions.

CHAPTER 14

EAHCA (Education for All Handicapped Children Act); IDEA (Individuals with Disabilities Education Act)

SHAWN S. SIDHU

HENDRICK HUDSON BOARD OF EDUCATION V. ROWLEY, 458 U.S. 176 (1982)

Link to case: http://caselaw.lp.findlaw.com/scripts/getcase.pl?navby=case&court=us&vol=458&page=176

Question: Does the EAHCA require schools to provide handicapped children "an opportunity to achieve full potential commensurate with the opportunity provided to other children?"

Answer: No.

Amy Rowley was a hearing-impaired student in New York who was otherwise bright and good at lip reading. Her parents, who were also both hearing impaired, met with the school a year prior to her starting kindergarten to discuss her education. In preparation, the school incorporated some technologies to help communicate with the family, and some staff members attended a course in sign language. Because Amy had some minimal residual hearing and was able to read lips well, she had success in kindergarten with the use of an FM transmitter. Prior to first grade, an Individualized Education Plan (IEP) meeting was held recommending placement in a mainstream classroom. The school also agreed to provide individual tutoring for 1 hour per day and speech therapy 3 hours a week. Amy's parents wanted her to also have a qualified sign language interpreter for all of her academic endeavors. The school ultimately found this unnecessary because the student was doing well academically and functioning relatively independently. A district court and the U.S. Court of Appeals for the Second Circuit sided with Amy's parents until the case was petitioned to the U.S. Supreme Court by the Hendrick Hudson Central School District. The Court ultimately reversed the judgment of the two lower courts, citing that the "free and appropriate public education" standard mandates that schools provide services that "permit the child to benefit from the instruction." The Court went on to write that the services provided by the school district "offered her [Amy] an educational opportunity substantially equal to that provided her non-handicapped classmates." While additional services may have allowed Amy to "maximally benefit" from her educational setting, she had achieved academic success with the services already in place.

IRVING INDEPENDENT SCHOOL DISTRICT V. TATRO, 468 U.S. 883 (1984)

Link to case: http://caselaw.lp.findlaw.com/scripts/getcase.pl?navby=case&court=us&vol=468&page=883

Question: Is a child with spina bifida entitled to urinary catheterization during school hours under the EAHCA?

Answer: Yes.

Amber Tatro was an 8-year-old student attending Irving Independent School District at the time of the case. She had spina bifida, which resulted in orthopedic pathology and speech abnormalities. The student was also unable to voluntarily empty her bladder completely at regular intervals due to a neurogenic bladder. Failure to empty her bladder would have resulted in damage to her kidneys, and therefore she required assistance emptying her bladder every 3 to 4 hours via clean intermittent catheterization (CIC). The catheterization procedure was a simple one that did not require medical training to complete, but rather could be completed by school nurses or any other trained adult. At Amber's IEP meeting, her parents requested that the school provide CIC services while Amber was at school; however, the school district refused on the grounds that CIC is a medical procedure and therefore should not be performed by school staff. Amber's parents brought the matter before the district court and state board of education. The district court ruled in favor of the school district, arguing that CIC is not a "related service" under the Education of the Handicapped Act because it was not directly related to education. The Court of Appeals for the Fifth Circuit reversed the ruling of the district court, stating that CIC was indeed a "related service," and further argued that not providing this service excluded Amber from access to basic educational services. The school district then brought the matter before the U.S. Supreme Court, which ruled in favor of Amber. The Court ruled that CIC is a "supportive service" without which Amber would not have been able to attend school, much less access special education. It ruled that CIC was not a "medical service," defined as "services provided by a licensed physician," because CIC can be performed by a school nurse or any other qualified adult who has received appropriate training.

CHAPTER 15

Questions on Child and Adolescent Issues

QUESTIONS

1. The Education for All Handicapped Children Act (now known as the Individuals with Disabilities Education Act [IDEA]) was based on the expectation that all disabled children should have which of the following?
   A. Tuition waivers for more individualized private schools
   B. A free and appropriate public education
   C. Placement in a special education classroom
   D. Institutionalized education for the severely disabled
   E. Access to specialized nonpublic schools

2. The minimum standard of proof for the termination of parental rights is:
   A. Beyond a reasonable doubt
   B. Preponderance of the evidence
   C. Clear and convincing evidence
   D. More likely than not

3. In *Graham v. Florida*, the U.S. Supreme Court ruled that:
   A. The sentence of "life without parole" is prohibited for individuals who committed any offenses under the age of 18.
   B. The sentence of "life without parole" for individuals who commit nonhomicide crimes when under the age of 18 violates the Fourteenth Amendment's requirement for equal protection.

C. The sentence of "life without parole" for individuals who commit nonhomicide offenses when under the age of 18 violates the Eighth Amendment's prohibition on cruel and unusual punishment.
D. The sentence of "life without parole" for individuals who commit nonhomicide offenses when under the age of 18 violates both the Eighth and Fourteenth Amendments.

4. The importance of protecting psychotherapist–patient privilege is maintained by the following rationale:
   A. The protection of privacy in a psychotherapist–patient relationship is thought to be important in establishing therapeutic alliance and to facilitate engagement in treatment.
   B. Law enforcement needs supersede psychotherapist–patient privilege.
   C. Mandated reporting of sexual abuse has a higher priority than reporting neglect.
   D. Police can compel physicians and therapists to testify in cases of sexual abuse involving minors.
   E. Psychotherapists must weigh maintaining patient privilege when public safety concerns exist around sexual abuse.

5. In the United States, execution is allowed for:
   A. Juveniles under the age of 18
   B. Mentally retarded individuals
   C. Individuals with severe psychotic disorders
   D. Individuals who are so impaired that they do not understand why they are being executed

6. An 11-year-old student with chronic renal failure and end-stage kidney disease requires hemodialysis multiple times weekly. The patient's parents would like the child to have this service provided at school so as to minimally disrupt the educational process. Which of the following best describes the school's level of responsibility to perform the procedure based on the precedent set by *Irving Independent School District v. Tatro*?
   A. Transport the student to and from the procedure.
   B. Provide funding for the procedure.
   C. The school has no responsibility for the procedure.
   D. Send a private tutor with the student to the procedure.
   E. Perform the procedure at the school.

7. The principle utilized in *Painter v. Bannister* for the determination of child custody was:
   A. The tender years doctrine
   B. The best interests of the child
   C. Least detrimental alternative
   D. Primary caregiver standard

8. Juvenile courts:
   A. Have been a fixture in the United States since colonial times
   B. Are a relatively recent invention, with the first juvenile court appearing in 1899 in Illinois
   C. Like criminal courts operate under the parens patriae principle
   D. Have always functioned similarly with respect to the roles and educations of attorneys and judges

9. The holdings of the U.S. Supreme Court in *Santosky v. Kramer* as they pertain to the termination of parental rights include:
   A. The primary interest of the state in parental termination hearings is the best interests of the child.
   B. While parents have an interest in preserving the family, the state has no such interest.
   C. There are shared interests in an accurate and just decision at fact-finding proceedings, and the near-equal allocation of risk between parents and the state is unconstitutional.
   D. The natural parents were not negligent, and the Santosky children should not have been removed.

10. When federal and state laws differ about a disabled student's entitlement to services, which of the following best summarizes the appropriate approach?
    A It is permissible to follow the state law if it has fewer mandates than the federal law.
    B. Both laws must be put before a legal professional who is an expert in case law to establish the best next step.
    C. The parents can list their preference with regard to which law is followed based on the subsequent services to be provided.
    D. The federal and the state laws both apply when the state requirements extend beyond the federal.
    E. The school district can choose the law that seems more applicable as long as it cites the reason for doing so.

11. Among the constitutional rights afforded juvenile defendants after *In re Gault* are:
    A. The right to an appeal
    B. The right to a jury trial
    C. The right to counsel
    D. The right to bail and a speedy trial

12. Implications of *Santosky v. Kramer* for children include:
    A. Child protective services will have a more difficult time investigating neglect and abuse allegations.
    B. Some children will not be removed from abusive or neglectful homes because it is more difficult to find clear and convincing evidence of abuse or neglect.
    C. More funding was made available for child protective service agencies around the country.
    D. Child protective services are able to remove children from abusive or neglectful homes more easily and efficiently than before.

13. Concepts underlying the philosophy of the juvenile court include:
    A. Closed proceedings and sealed records prevent discovery of procedural irregularities.
    B. The disposition should fit the offender rather than the offense in the interest of rehabilitation.
    C. Punishment as an extension of just desserts.
    D. Punishment is reserved for only the most severe and heinous of crimes, such as rape and murder.

14. A physician evaluates a child and is concerned about the potential for child abuse. The physician makes a report to child protective services, and the case is ultimately closed when no suspicious activity is found. The parents feel humiliated by the allegation and sue the physician for defamation and a violation of privacy. Which of the following most accurately represents the legal stance regarding this matter?
    A. Courts in most states tend to prioritize the rights of parents, and the physician is potentially liable.
    B. States vary greatly on this issue, and there is little national consensus on the matter.

C. The outcomes of these cases are most dependent on the testimony of the child.
D. Physicians who report in good faith are generally immune from liability for any damages.
E. Parents are typically not allowed to bring suits against physicians for violations of privacy.

15. A clear and convincing standard for the termination of parental rights is justified because:
    A. Parental termination proceedings resemble criminal trials, and parents who face removal are often poor and uneducated and do not have the resources to oppose the state; therefore, it is more likely with a preponderance of the evidence standard that errors will be made.
    B. Parents have the right to reasonably discipline their children.
    C. DSS does not give parents assistance in reestablishing a weakened parent-child bond.
    D. A liberty issue is not at stake.

16. In *DeShaney v. Winnebago*, the main thrust of the ruling is based on the following principle:
    A. Due process protections are the foundation for mandated child abuse reporting statutes.
    B. The state has a duty to provide youth with adequate protection from all forms of abuse from parents.
    C. The state has a duty to provide youth with protection from harm from state agents.
    D. The Due Process Clause protects citizens against state actions and those of private citizens.

17. In *Graham v. Florida*, the Supreme Court cited which of the following in support of its opinion?
    A. Juveniles are immature and have an underdeveloped sense of responsibility.
    B. Most jurisdictions that technically allow juveniles to receive a life sentence without parole only rarely impose such a sentence.
    C. Juveniles are more capable of change than adults.
    D. All of the above.

18. Which of the following is correct with respect to the Iowa Supreme Court's custody decision in *Painter v. Bannister*?
    A. Security and stability in the home are more important than intellectual stimulation in the development of a child.

B. A parent's or caretaker's philosophy and way of life "within normal and proper limits" are irrelevant with respect to the determination of custody.
C. The expert testimony of the child psychiatrist was afforded negligible weight.
D. The child's relationship with his grandfather, which was stronger than that with his father, received little attention in the decision.

19. Which of the following is correct about sentencing guidelines for a 15-year-old convicted of capital murder in adult court?
    A. The fact-finder is required to impose a minimum sentence of life without parole, although the death penalty can be considered.
    B. The fact-finder is required to impose a minimum sentence of life without parole but cannot consider the death penalty.
    C. The fact-finder cannot sentence the defendant to life without parole.
    D. The fact-finder must consider the impact of youth when imposing a sentence.
    E. A 15-year-old cannot be tried in adult court.

20. Which of the following best justifies a breach in physician–patient confidentiality in cases of suspected child abuse?
    A. Justice for the alleged perpetrator
    B. The safety of the patient at risk
    C. Prevention of professional liability
    D. The safety of the public at large
    E. Physician acting as an agent of the state

ANSWERS

1. **B**
The EAHCA mandated that all handicapped children receive a "free appropriate public education." This term has continued to be applied in educational settings and, although vague, is the basis for many of today's educational standards. While some children spend time in special education classrooms and others go to specialized nonpublic schools, these do not apply to all disabled students and depend on individual and local district resources.

2. **C**
The minimum standard of proof for the termination of parental rights is clear and convincing evidence. In *Santosky v. Kramer*, the U.S.

Supreme Court noted that parents faced with the irrevocable dissolution of their parental rights have a greater need for procedural protections than do parents resisting state involvement in ongoing family matters, such as temporarily removing children secondary to neglect.

3. **C**

    In *Roper v. Simmons* (2005), the U.S. Supreme Court held that executing individuals under age 18 at the time of the offense was a violation of the Eighth Amendment's prohibition against cruel and unusual punishment. In *Graham v. Florida*, the majority opinion of the Court reaffirmed their reasoning, holding that juveniles were immature and therefore less culpable and less deserving of the most severe punishments. Neither case prohibited imposing the sentence of life without parole on individuals who commit murder before the age of 18.

4. **A**

    Law enforcement needs do not necessarily compel breeches in doctor–patient or psychotherapist–patient confidentiality. Regardless of the type, mandated reporters should report all child maltreatment to the appropriate authority if a reasonable suspicion exists. While a psychotherapist is indeed a mandated reporter of child abuse, the protection of privilege stems from the need to maintain treatment engagement and a therapeutic alliance, not public safety interests.

5. **C**

    The Constitution does not prohibit the death penalty in severely mentally ill individuals, even if they are psychotic, as long as the individual understands the reason for his or her imminent execution (*Panetti v. Quarterman*, 551 U.S. 930 [2007]). The Supreme Court in *Panetti* declined to define what level of rational understanding a death row inmate needed, indicating that it hoped that psychiatric expert testimony would shed light on whether an inmate's delusions were so severe as to render him or her incompetent to be executed.

6. **C**

    Given that hemodialysis is a complicated medical procedure that employs the use of a dialysis machine and requires specialized training to administer, it would be considered a "medical service" rather than a "supportive service," and the school would not have any additional responsibility beyond common courtesy (observing the patient, alerting parents and authorities if the patient does not appear to be doing well, etc.). Funding should come from the patient's insurance or public

7. **B**

In *Painter v. Bannister*, the Iowa Supreme Court concluded that remaining in the secure and stable custody of grandparents, rather than the unstable, but potentially more intellectually stimulating, custody of the father served the best interests of the child. Most jurisdictions determine custody on the basis of the best interests of the child standard, although considerable judicial discretion is allowed.

8. **B**

The first juvenile court appeared in 1899 in Chicago, Illinois, and the concept grew in popularity. In juvenile court, the state as parens patriae would act as an advocate of youths, rather than as an adversary, and provide them with the help and treatment they required to overcome their youthful misdeeds. Due process was not considered to be necessary because the state was acting on behalf of the juvenile and therefore protection was unnecessary. Formal rules and procedures might hamper the court's mission and prescriptive "treatments." Prior to *Gault*, the key players in the juvenile court were social workers, mental health professionals, and probation officers. There was little law, therefore little need for attorneys, and many of the judges were not legally trained. The most important question revolved around amenability to treatment.

9. **C**

Justice Blackmun in the majority opinion wrote that the Court expressed no opinion regarding the merits of the Santoskys' claims regarding their fitness for parenting the children who had been removed and noted that at "a hearing conducted under a constitutionally proper standard" (clear and convincing evidence, rather than preponderance of the evidence), "they may or may not prevail." The Court vacated the judgment of the New York Appellate Division and remanded the case for further proceedings. The "best interests of the child" standard was more clearly articulated in *Painter v. Bannister*.

10. **D**

With regard to the education of handicapped students, federal law sets a bare minimally acceptable standard. Many states may extend regulations beyond this bare minimum, but state law may not undercut the minimal standard set by the U.S. Congress or Supreme Court.

11. **C**

    In re Gault's decision held that juveniles had the right to notice of charges, to counsel, to confrontation and cross-examination of witnesses, and to privilege against self-incrimination. Juveniles in juvenile court do not have the right to an appeal, a jury trial, a transcript of the proceedings, or the right to a speedy trial. Youths who are tried in adult court do have these rights.

12. **B**

    Some child advocates have noted that by making termination of parental rights more difficult by raising the burden of proof, the Supreme Court decision in *Santosky v. Kramer* created a presumption against termination of parental rights, and that children have rights that do not necessary coincide with those of their parents or the state. The higher burden and proof may result in the already overstretched agencies charged with investigating abuse and neglect to have inadequate evidence to meet the increased burden; hence more children will remain in neglectful homes.

13. **B**

    Proceedings are closed and records sealed in juvenile court to avoid stigma and are in keeping with the benevolent nature of the court. Because the focus of the juvenile court is on rehabilitation and treatment rather than punishment, the disposition is tailored to the offender rather than the offense.

14. **D**

    While all of the answer choices in this question could technically be correct depending on the specific situation, the best answer is that doctors are generally protected when making decisions in the best interest of the child. Physicians may be held liable if the reporting is malicious, antagonistic, or otherwise unfounded. However, the law clearly favors reporting suspected abuse over withholding suspicions due to concerns about parental confidentiality. Potential penalties for not reporting suspected abuse are significantly greater than violations of confidentiality.

15. **A**

    In its decision, the U.S. Supreme Court noted that there was a liberty issue at stake in *Santosky v. Kramer*, and more substantial than the loss of money or property, where the standard of proof is preponderance of the evidence. The Court noted that the parents' interest in a termination proceeding is major (the loss of their children and family), and there is substantial risk of error involved if the standard used is preponderance of the evidence. Additionally, the government interest in favoring the preponderance of the evidence standard is slight. The Court's opinion also reflected the difficulty that poor, uneducated parents may have in mounting a defense against "[t]he State's ability to assemble its case" and referred to the state's "unusual ability to structure evidence," increasing the "risk of an erroneous fact finding," noting that DSS sought court orders denying the Santoskys visitation with their children, which if successful would have put them out of compliance with the Family Court Act's requirement for maintaining contact with their children.

16. **C**

In *DeShaney v. Winnebago*, the court ruled that the Due Process Clause protects citizens against state action but *not* against the actions of private citizens. The state has a duty to provide youths with protection from harm from state agents only. State child abuse reporting requirements preempt physician–patient privilege. *Landeros v. Flood* relates to establishing battered child syndrome and is a foundational case in establishing mandated reporting of child abuse and neglect.

17. **D**

In *Graham v. Florida* the Supreme Court utilized the same reasoning as in *Roper v. Simmons*. These include (1) juveniles' lack of maturity and underdeveloped sense of responsibility; (2) their increased susceptibility to negative influences and outside pressures, including peer pressure; and (3) their more malleable personalities, which are "not as well formed."

18. **A**

While some of the biases revealed by the Iowa Supreme Court in *Painter v. Bannister* are often quoted, including his "artsy" father's "bohemian lifestyle," the court's opinion clearly indicates that the judges attempted to thoughtfully consider what was in the child's best interests and had an appreciation of the fact that the "divergent life patterns" of the father "seem[ed] to represent alternative normal adaptations." They attempted to contextualize the differences in lifestyle and the facts of the case as they applied to Mark Bannister. As is often the case in today's child custody disputes, the opinion of the expert witness in this case was given considerable weight. However, it is interesting to note that the trial court, which awarded custody to the father, dismissed the testimony of the expert, in part because it was "dismissive" of the role of the natural father. One of the factors given weight by the Supreme Court was that the psychologist opined that it was "very evident" that Mark considered his grandfather to be his father figure.

19. **D**

According to *Miller v. Alabama*, trial courts must consider the contribution of youth (including developmental immaturity and diminished culpability) when sentencing juveniles who have been convicted of serious crimes (e.g., murder). Mandatory sentencing guidelines of life without parole for juveniles violate the Eighth Amendment, and therefore (A) and (B) are incorrect. However, there is still room for the fact-finder to sentence a juvenile to life without parole if the factors of youth have been considered; (C) is therefore incorrect. Answer (E) is incorrect because adolescents in many jurisdictions can be tried in adult court for certain crimes.

20. **B**

Answers B, C, and E are all potential justifications for physicians to beach confidentiality. For example, when quarantining an infectious patient, physicians are protecting the public at large and acting as an agent of the state. In these cases, the safety of individual patients may even take a back seat to that of the general public. However, in the case of child abuse, a breach of confidentiality is specifically intended to protect the patient. Preventing liability is secondary to patient safety issues.

SECTION IV

Tort Law

The cases in this section address mental health–related civil law. Specific topics include workers' compensation, the Americans with Disabilities Act (ADA), negligence, insurance, and sexual harassment. Each of these areas is important for the practicing forensic psychiatrist. For forensic practitioners engaged as experts, an understanding of how the law thinks about mental or emotional damage and the concepts of negligence and duty as they relate to psychiatric injury is critical. Similarly, familiarity with what constitutes sexual harassment is the necessary foundation for understanding the role of the forensic practitioner in such cases. The ADA and insurance cases raise both litigation-specific issues and policy-level considerations that affect the general delivery of mental health care. Each state, for example, continues to maintain an "Olmstead list" of individuals deemed appropriate for less than a hospital level of care, who should be discharged as rapidly as is reasonable.

Some of these cases, particularly in the health insurance chapter, may seem relatively removed from most of the readers' daily practice and are generally considered to contain some of the most dense and challenging language to interpret. However, as of this writing, they remain on the ABPN list of cases that should be reviewed for the initial certification exam in forensic psychiatry. In light of the current climate around health insurance coverage in the United States, they are also useful in understanding the Supreme Court's historical discussions on this topic.

CHAPTER 16

ADA/Disability

HOWARD FORMAN

CARTER V. GENERAL MOTORS, 106 N.W. 2D 105 (1960)

Link to case: http://scholar.google.com/scholar_case?case=1155130287709691700

Question: Are emotional disabilities compensable under workers' compensation even if they do not result from a direct physical injury or a single mentally disturbing event (e.g., seeing a coworker crushed to death)?

Answer: Yes.

James Carter was employed by General Motors (GM) and developed psychosis. Mr. Carter sought workers' compensation benefits. Medical testimony by Mr. Carter's treating psychiatrist stated that his psychosis resulted from emotional pressure encountered during the course of his daily work activities (assembly line work). The treating psychiatrist testified that, at some point, Mr. Carter's psychotic symptoms completely resolved, but that he could not return to the same type of employment because the pressures of the job might lead him to become psychotic again. The Michigan Workman's Compensation Appeals Board granted Mr. Carter benefits even though the psychosis resulted from "emotional pressures" rather than from a "single fortuitous event" such as a workplace accident. Also, the board granted benefits on an ongoing basis, having found that Mr. Carter could not return to work because of the risk of the return of psychotic symptoms. General Motors appealed the decision to the Michigan State Supreme Court. The court affirmed that although Mr. Carter only became psychotic while working at GM because of normal daily pressures combined with Mr. Carter's "predisposition to the development of a schizophrenic process," he was entitled to workers' compensation during the period of his psychosis. The Michigan State Supreme Court reversed the decision that Mr. Carter was entitled to ongoing benefits once his psychosis had resolved because at that point he would return to being a person with the "predisposition" to develop psychosis.

BRAGDON V. ABBOTT, 524 U.S. 624 (1998)

Link to case: http://scholar.google.com/scholar_case?case=11295524924367699420

Question: Is HIV status a disability as defined by the ADA?

Answer: Yes.

Sidney Abbott had asymptomatic HIV and went to her dentist to have a cavity filled. The dentist, Dr. Randon Bragdon, refused to perform the procedure unless it was done in a hospital, claiming that any other setting would pose a risk to him. Although Dr. Bragdon stated that he would not charge extra for his services, Ms. Abbott would have to pay any costs related to the use of the hospital's facility. The ADA defines a health care provider's office as a "place of public accommodation" covered by the act, but protections from the ADA may be set aside when the disabled individual "poses a direct threat to the health or safety of others." Ms. Abbott sued Dr. Bragdon on the ground that he violated the ADA because he discriminated against her on the basis of HIV, which she claimed met criteria as an ADA disability since it is a "physical impairment" that "substantially limits" a "major life activity" (i.e., her ability to reproduce and bear children). The district court and the U.S. Court of Appeals for the First Circuit both ruled in favor of Ms. Abbott, reasoning that (1) HIV infection (even when asymptomatic) is a disability, and (2) according to standards promulgated by the ADA, her HIV did not present any direct threat to Dr. Bragdon's health in his office. The U.S. Supreme Court agreed with the lower court decisions that HIV is a disability but remanded the case to the appeals court for consideration of whether Dr. Bragdon had a reasonable claim that performing the procedure placed him at risk.

PENNSYLVANIA V. YESKEY, 524 U.S. 206 (1998)

Link to case: http://scholar.google.com/scholar_case?case=3291537490094626018

Question: Does the ADA apply to people who are incarcerated in state prisons?

Answer: Yes.

Ronald Yeskey was sentenced to 18 to 36 months in Pennsylvania State Prison for drunken driving, escape, and resisting arrest. The sentencing court recommended that he be placed in Pennsylvania's motivational boot camp for first-time offenders. If Mr. Yeskey completed the boot camp successfully, he would only be incarcerated for a total of 6 months and then paroled. Mr. Yeskey was denied admission to the boot camp because he suffered from hypertension. He subsequently sued Pennsylvania's Department of Corrections, claiming it had violated the ADA by denying him the opportunity to participate in a program that could shorten his incarceration. The district court dismissed Yeskey's claim on the grounds that state prisons are not subject to the ADA. The U.S. Court of Appeals for the Third Circuit reversed this decision, holding that state prisons are in fact subject to the ADA. Pennsylvania appealed to the U.S. Supreme Court and supported its appeal in part with the language of the ADA, which states that denying disabled people "benefits" is prohibited. The state argued that prison is not intended to benefit the inmate. The U.S. Supreme Court affirmed the appellate decision and said that Mr. Yeskey was indeed entitled to protection from discrimination despite being an inmate.

OLMSTEAD V. ZIMRING, 527 U.S. 581 (1999)

Link to case: http://caselaw.lp.findlaw.com/scripts/getcase.pl?navby=case&court=us&vol=527&page=581#section1

Question: Does continued confinement of individuals with mental disabilities in hospitals beyond their clinical need for that level of care constitute discrimination under the ADA?

Answer: Yes.

Tommy Olmstead was the commissioner of the Georgia Department of Resources. Jonathan Zimring was a guardian ad litem for L.C., a mentally retarded woman with schizophrenia. L.C. was admitted to Georgia

Regional Hospital for treatment of her psychiatric illness. After a period of inpatient treatment, it was determined by treating clinicians at the hospital that L.C. could safely be treated in a community-based program; however, she remained in the hospital pending placement in an appropriate outpatient program. She sued for relief pursuant to the ADA, arguing that her continued confinement was discriminatory in that she was precluded from access to the community equal to that of those without her disability. The district court granted partial judgment for Zimring, partially upheld by the U.S. Court of Appeals for the Eleventh Circuit. It remanded the case for reconsideration of Georgia's argument about the resource burden of providing community-based treatment in a timely way. The U.S. Supreme Court agreed with Zimring that "unjustified segregation of persons with disabilities is a form of discrimination" and held that "states are required to place persons with mental disabilities in community settings when the State's treatment professionals have determined that community placement is appropriate...is not opposed by the affected individual, and the placement can be reasonably accommodated, taking into account the resources available to the State and the needs of others with mental disabilities." In appreciation of Georgia's concerns, the Court held that a state need not immediately transfer everyone to a community-based program but must have a mechanism by which people who are eligible to be transferred can be within a reasonable amount of time.

TOYOTA V. WILLIAMS, 534 U.S. 184 (2002)

Link to case: http://scholar.google.com/scholar_case?case=3382304874478067867

Question: Does a disability that limits only specific work-related tasks qualify as a disability under the ADA?

Answer: No.

Ella Williams was a Toyota employee who suffered from carpal tunnel syndrome. Ms. Williams sued Toyota under the ADA, alleging that Toyota did not make "reasonable accommodations" for her disability. Toyota argued that carpal tunnel syndrome did not qualify as a disability because it did not substantially limit any of Ms. Williams's major life activities. The district court ruled in favor of Toyota, but the U.S. Court of Appeals for the Sixth Circuit reversed and ruled that Ms. Williams's inability to continue her work as a manual laborer represented an inability to perform a "major life activity." The U.S. Supreme Court reversed the appeals court decision, holding that the appellate court did not apply the proper standard for defining a disability because it failed to ask whether the condition prevented or restricted Ms. Williams from performing tasks that are of central importance to most people's daily lives. The Supreme Court held, "Merely having an impairment does not make one disabled for purposes of the ADA. Claimants also need to demonstrate that the impairment limits a major life activity." "Major life activities" refer to those activities that are central to daily life.

HARGRAVE V. VERMONT, 340 F.3D 27 (2003)

Link to case: http://scholar.google.com/scholar_case?case=6285186011968139170

Question: Does a validly executed durable power of attorney, which specifies preferred treatment alternatives, carry the same weight for individuals hospitalized for mental illnesses as for those without mental illness?

Answer: Yes.

Vermont law allowed individuals to execute a durable power of attorney (DPOA) for health care decisions in case they become incapacitated. Nancy Hargrave was civilly committed to Vermont State Hospital. She had previously executed a DPOA forbidding her agent from consenting to "any and all anti-psychotic, neuroleptic, psychotropic, or psychoactive medication." The hospital medicated Ms. Hargrave in a nonemergent situation. She sued, claiming that her DPOA was ignored because of her mental illness and that her mental illness rendered her disabled and thereby protected by the ADA. Vermont Act 114, which allowed the state to medicate a civilly committed individual even if the individual had a DPOA refusing treatment, had no corresponding mechanism for medication over objection for people who were only physically ill. The state argued that no corresponding mechanism was necessary, since mental illness in an involuntarily committed individual posed a "significant risk" and was not due protection by the ADA. The district court granted summary judgment in favor of Ms. Hargrave, stating that Vermont Act 114 singled out the mentally ill for discrimination and thus violated the ADA; the U.S. Court of Appeals for the Second Circuit upheld the holding.

U.S. V. GEORGIA, 546 U.S. 151 (2006)

Link to case: http://caselaw.lp.findlaw.com/scripts/getcase.pl?navby=case&court=us&vol=546&page=151

Question: Can a disabled inmate in a state prison sue the state under Title II of the ADA?

Answer: Yes.

Tony Goodman, a paraplegic inmate at Georgia State Prison in Reisdville, sued the State of Georgia, claiming that he was being discriminated against because of his disability in violation of the ADA. He alleged that during his time in prison he was confined 23 hours a day in a cell so narrow he could not turn his wheelchair around. He also alleged that he was denied access to programming, medical services, and needed assistance with bathing and toileting. Georgia argued that it did not have to accommodate Mr. Goodman because the ADA violated its state sovereignty under the Eleventh Amendment, which prohibits the federal government from impinging on states' autonomy except as specifically provided in the Constitution. The district court dismissed the case, stating that "state sovereign immunity" barred Title II ADA claims. The U.S. Court of Appeals for the Eleventh Circuit agreed about the ADA claims but reversed the decision based on Eighth Amendment claims. The U.S. Supreme Court then granted certiorari "to consider whether Title II of the ADA validly abrogates state sovereign immunity" against claims related to Fourteenth Amendment (equal protection) violations and therefore allows a state prisoner to sue for money damages. The Court concluded that Congress had the "power to enforce, by appropriate legislation" the constitutional guarantee of equal protection across states and that therefore the ADA created a private cause of action against states for conduct that violates the Fourteenth Amendment.

CHAPTER 17

Emotional Harm

AMAR MEHTA

DILLON V. LEGG, 441 P.2D 912 (1968)

Link to case: http://scholar.google.com/scholar_case?case=1779068908894362158

Question: Does a person who suffers emotional injury but was not exposed to actual physical injury have standing to sue for negligence?

Answer: Yes.

In 1964, Margery Dillon was crossing a street several yards behind two of her daughters. David Legg was driving a car that struck and killed one daughter. Ms. Dillon filed suit seeking compensation for her deceased daughter, as well as damages for herself and her surviving daughter. Mr. Legg moved for a summary judgment on Ms. Dillon's claim of emotional suffering, and it was granted by the Superior Court on the grounds that Ms. Dillon could not have feared for her own safety because she was not in the "zone of danger," or an area within which she was at risk of actual physical harm. The Supreme Court of California reversed the decision on appeal, describing "the hopeless artificiality" of the rule by pointing out that "the area of those exposed to *emotional* injury" is much broader, and "no distinction can be drawn between physical and emotional injury." The court maintained a standard of "reasonable foreseeability" and offered guidelines to take into account factors such as whether a plaintiff was near the scene, whether his or her shock was the result of directly observing the accident at the time, and whether he or she was closely related to the direct victim.

THING V. LA CHUSA, 771 P.2D 814 (1989)

Link to case: http://scholar.google.com/scholar_case?case=4005949371237649225

Question: Is the "foreseeability" standard established by *Dillon v. Legg* too expansive?

Answer: Yes.

In 1980, James La Chusa was driving his car when he hit a boy named John Thing. John's sister quickly told their mother, Maria, who rushed over to the road and saw her injured son. Ms. Thing then sued Mr. La Chusa for emotional harm, alleging that his negligence caused the injury to John and was proximately responsible for her distress. Mr. La Chusa successfully requested a summary judgment from the trial court on the grounds that Ms. Thing had not witnessed the accident herself. The appellate court reversed that judgment, giving legal standing back to Ms. Thing. Finally, the Supreme Court of California ruled that the trial court had been correct, and that Ms. Thing could not establish such a claim. It laid out strict conditions necessary to recover for the negligent infliction of emotional distress, which had become too expansive and confusing since *Dillon v. Legg*. Instead of following a broad "foreseeability" standard, a plaintiff had to be closely related to the injury victim, had to be present for and aware of the "injury-producing event" at the time, and had to have suffered more emotional distress than a "disinterested witness."

CHAPTER 18

Health Insurance

BRYAN C. SHELBY, MERRILL ROTTER,
AND ELIZABETH FORD

AETNA V. MCCABE, 556 F. SUPP. 1342 (1983)

Link to case: http://scholar.google.com/scholar_case?case=14176085046214731005

Question: Is an insurance carrier responsible for covering alleged malpractice involving sexual relations between a physician and patient?

Answer: Yes.

Aetna, a malpractice insurance carrier, sought a declaration of noncoverage, arguing that the sexual relationship between Dr. Donald McCabe and Ms. Gale Greenberg (1) "did not arise out of professional services" and (2) constituted an "intentional tort" (as opposed to an accident); thus, punitive damages should not be paid by the insurer. Ms. Greenberg was in treatment with Dr. McCabe for asthma and anxiety. Dr. McCabe provided therapy and medication that was "either illicit or 'contraindicated.'" Their sexual relationship began after 6 months, and they eventually lived together. Dr. McCabe continued to prescribe medication throughout their relationship. At trial, there was testimony that Dr. McCabe's treatment and "mishandling" of the transference fell below professional standards. The jury found in favor of Aetna. On appeal, the court found that Aetna had represented Dr. McCabe throughout the trial and had not made the professional services argument, and so could not now argue that the sexual relationship was not covered by the policy. The court further noted that the policy did not explicitly exclude "intentional" behavior from coverage. Finally, the court found that Dr. McCabe should not be able to shield himself from the pain of punitive damages through insurance, and so those could not be covered by the policy.

MAZZA V. MEDICAL MUTUAL INSURANCE COMPANY OF NORTH CAROLINA, 311 N.C. 621 (1984)

Link to case: http://www.leagle.com/decision/1984536319SE2d217_1529

Question: Does public policy prohibit insurance coverage of punitive damages based on medical malpractice?

Answer: No.

Dr. Robert Huffaker was the treating psychiatrist of Jeffery Mazza, who alleged that Dr. Huffaker engaged in sexual intercourse with Mr. Mazza's estranged wife and abandoned him at a vulnerable time during treatment. Mr. Mazza sued Dr. Huffaker, claiming medical malpractice and other grounds for relief. Dr. Huffaker had an insurance policy in effect issued by Medical Mutual. At trial, Mr. Mazza was awarded $102,000 in compensatory and $500,000 in punitive damages, and the court further issued a declaratory judgment that the insurance contract obligated Medical Mutual to pay. On appeal, the North Carolina Supreme Court held that, while North Carolina law was silent on this question, other state courts had found that insurance contracts could be held to cover punitive damages. The court upheld Dr. Huffaker's acts as medical negligence and not as intentional acts. Furthermore, the court stated that punitive damages are available for acts that are not just intentional but also "wanton, reckless, malicious or oppressive." The terms of the Medical Mutual insurance contract were interpreted to be broad enough to cover the punitive damages based on Dr. Huffaker's medical negligence.

WICKLINE V. STATE, 192 CAL. APP. 3D 1630 (1987)

Link to case: http://scholar.google.com/scholar_case?case=15274898154834148181

Question: Did California's third-party payer owe damages for harm caused by the application of a cost-containment program that affected a treating doctor's medical judgment?

Answer: No.

Lois Wickline was diagnosed with Leriche's syndrome, which could only be treated surgically. Mrs. Wickline's health insurance, Medi-Cal, authorized surgery and 10 days of hospitalization for her condition. She underwent several surgeries over those 10 days. Her treating physicians determined she needed 8 more days of hospitalization, but Medi-Cal's reviewers denied this request, and her treating doctors did not protest or appeal this decision. She was discharged but returned to the hospital with complications that resulted in the amputation of her right leg. Mrs. Wickline sued Med-Cal for damages. The jury found for Mrs. Wickline. On appeal, the California Court of Appeals held that Medi-Cal, as the third-party payer, was not liable because the treating physician went along with the shortened length of stay. Mrs. Wickline's doctors never protested or requested an administrative appeal of Medi-Cal's initial decision. Although the court did not decide in Mrs. Wickline's favor in this case, it did note that third-party payers may be held liable in instances of design defects in the cost containment system or arbitrary decisions regarding care reimbursement.

WILSON V. BLUE CROSS OF SOUTHERN CALIFORNIA, 222 CAL. APP. 3D 660 (1990)

Link to case: http://scholar.google.com/scholar_case?case=16670556625035342312

Question: As a matter of law, are there triable issues of fact against an insurance company medical review if the attending physician did not make an appeal?

Answer: Yes.

Howard Wilson was admitted to a hospital for psychiatric treatment. His treating doctor believed he needed a 3- to 4-week inpatient admission. Ten days after admission, however, the patient's insurance company would not pay for any further inpatient care. Unable to self-pay, Mr. Wilson was discharged. Three weeks later he committed suicide. His estate brought suit against the defendant insurance company, Blue Cross and Blue Shield, and the utilization review company, Western Medical. The companies successfully filed for summary judgment citing *Wickline*, but Mr. Wilson's estate appealed. On appeal, the California Court of Appeals stated that *Wickline* was not applicable in this case because the discharge in *Wickline* met the standard of care as a matter of law, did not involve an insurance contract, and involved a cost-containment program established by state law. Furthermore, even though the treating physician did not appeal the insurance company review and ultimately made the decision to discharge the patient, as had been dispositive in *Wickline*, it was not considered critical in this case. *Wickline*'s language, according to the court, was characterized as dicta and not controlling. Mr. Wilson's estate was granted permission to continue the lawsuit at trial.

CORCORAN V. UNITED HEALTHCARE, INC., 965 F.2D 1321 (1992)

Link to case: http://scholar.google.com/scholar_case?case=9371215507258986216

Question: Does the Employee Retirement Income Security Act of 1974 (ERISA), designed to provide government oversight of employee benefit plans, preempt state law malpractice claims brought by a beneficiary of an ERISA plan against the plan and utilization review company?

Answer: Yes.

Florence Corcoran was in the middle of her pregnancy when her obstetrician recommended she have complete bed rest until delivery. As her delivery date approached, her obstetrician admitted her to the hospital for fetal monitoring, but her company's insurance administrator, United Healthcare, would not certify a hospital stay, only home nursing care. While at home, when the home nurse was away, Mrs. Corcoran's fetus went into distress and died. Mrs. Corcoran filed suit in Louisiana state court alleging common law claims based on negligence against Blue Cross (the insurance company) and United (the administrative reviewing organization) for the loss of the fetus. The insurance companies removed the action to federal court on the grounds that it was preempted by ERISA. The federal court granted summary judgment, and Ms. Corcoran appealed to the U.S. Court of Appeals for the Fifth Circuit. In assessing whether the claims were preempted, the court reviewed the effects of the claims on an ERISA-governed plan and determined that while United made what appeared to be medical decisions, they were in fact determinations of benefits that made the case subject to ERISA rules. The court ruled that the only remedies available to Mrs. Corcoran would be those under ERISA.

NEW YORK STATE CONFERENCE OF BLUE CROSS AND BLUE SHIELD PLANS ET AL. V. TRAVELERS INSURANCE CO. ET AL., 514 U.S. 645 (1995)

Link to case: http://www.law.cornell.edu/supct/html/93-1408.ZS.html

Question: Was New York's statute requiring hospitals to collect surcharges from patients with certain health insurance coverage related enough to the administration of employee benefit plans to be preempted?

Answer: No.

New York State Public Health Law §2807 covers hospital billing rates for patient care not covered by Medicare. In 1993, patients covered by Medicaid, health maintenance organizations (HMOs), and Blue Cross/Blue Shield were billed at the diagnostic related group (DRG) rate for their conditions, but patients covered by commercial insurers, including Travelers, were billed for the DRG rate plus a 24% surcharge that went to the hospital and the state. HMOs were also variably charged up to 9% of monthly charges, payable to the state. Travelers et al., joined by several HMOs, sued New York State, joined by Blue Cross/Blue Shield, claiming that ERISA preempts surcharges for patients who have health insurance purchased by an ERISA plan. The district court granted summary judgment in favor of Travelers, stating that the surcharges were enough to significantly influence customers' ERISA plan choices and therefore were "related to" ERISA and preempted. The U.S. Court of Appeals for the Second Circuit affirmed the decision. The U.S. Supreme Court then heard the case and reversed. It found that the economic influence of these surcharges on ERISA plan purchasers was only indirect and was not enough to trigger preemption. The court was unimpressed with the cost uniformity argument, stating that reducing competition among insurance agencies was not the intention of Congress when it passed ERISA.

DUKES V. U.S. HEALTHCARE, INC., 57 F.3D 350 (1995)

Link to case: http://scholar.google.com/scholar_case?case=10046751704133491839

Question: Does ERISA preempt state malpractice actions against HMOs where medical care is arranged and provided by the HMO?

Answer: No.

This case involved two separate patient actions against the same HMO. The first patient, Darryl Dukes, was a member of the HMO U.S. Healthcare, through his employer-sponsored benefit plan. He sought treatment for several ailments from doctors employed by the HMO, but his condition worsened and he died. Ronald and Linda Visconti were parents of a child who was stillborn. Mrs. Viconti received her treatment through U.S. Healthcare and sued the company for medical malpractice. The HMO removed both cases to federal court, and the cases were consolidated on appeal. The U.S. Court of Appeals for the Third Circuit examined the nature of the claims related to the plaintiffs and found that they were neither claims to enforce their plan rights nor claims to past or future benefits. The court stated that these claims were about the quality of benefits provided and that since the HMOs were the actual arrangers and providers of medical care, the case was distinguished from *Corcoran*, where a third party simply reviewed the eligibility of benefits. The cases were remanded for further review at the trial court level.

AETNA V. DAVILA, 542 U.S. 200 (2004)

Link to case: http://scholar.google.com/scholar_case?case=4985418340165729455

Question: Does ERISA preempt claims for utilization review findings that adversely affect patient care?

Answer: Yes.

Juan Davila and Ruby Calad were participants and beneficiaries in their ERISA-regulated plans, Aetna Health Inc. and Cigna Healthcare, respectively. Mr. Davila alleged that Aetna refused to pay for Vioxx (rofecoxib) for his arthritis pain, and so he began taking Naprosyn (naproxen), which caused him a severe reaction and subsequent hospitalization. Ms. Calad underwent hospitalization, but CIGNA refused to pay for an extended hospital stay despite it being recommended by her treating physician. Ms. Calad experienced postsurgical complications and had to be readmitted to the hospital. Both Mr. Davila and Ms. Calad sued their respective plans under the Texas Health Care Liability Act (THCLA) in state court for medical malpractice. After the cases were removed to federal court, the participants appealed to remand to state court (the THCLA allowed for damages not available under federally regulated ERISA). The U.S. Court of Appeals for the Fifth Circuit agreed with the move back to state court, but the U.S. Supreme Court reversed and determined that

Mr. Davila's and Ms. Calad's claims were simply for a denial of benefits and were thus preempted under ERISA. Because the purpose of ERISA was to create a uniform system for regulation of employee benefit plans and benefit determinations, the court ruled that such claims fall under the scope of ERISA.

CHAPTER 19

Sexual Harassment

ANDREW P. LEVIN AND MERRILL ROTTER

MERITOR SAVINGS BANK V. VINSON, 477 U.S. 57 (1986)

Link to case: http://caselaw.lp.findlaw.com/scripts/getcase.pl?navby=case&court=us&vol=477&page=57

Question: Does a finding of sexual harassment require that the employee be subject to a quid pro quo linking the terms of employment to sexual favors?

Answer: No.

Over a 4-year period, Michelle Vinson worked her way up on merit from teller to assistant branch manager at Meritor Bank under the supervision of Sidney Taylor, one of the bank's vice presidents. After she was fired due to excessive sick leave, she filed suit under Title VII, claiming that she had been sexually harassed by Mr. Taylor (i.e., discriminated against on the basis of her sex). She alleged that Mr. Taylor made sexual advances to which she acquiesced for fear of losing her job and subjected her to demeaning fondling and comments in front of other employees. At trial the district court found that Ms. Vinson had not been the victim of sexual discrimination or sexual harassment because her relationship with Mr. Taylor was a voluntary one having nothing to do with her advancement or promotions. The U.S. Court of Appeals for the DC Circuit reversed, finding that sexual harassment includes the creation of a hostile or offensive work environment even when the terms and conditions of employment are not contingent on sexual favors (i.e., quid pro quo harassment). The U.S. Supreme

Court upheld the court of appeals ruling, affirming the Equal Employment Opportunity Commission's Guidance of 1980 that stated a "hostile environment" violates Title VII. The Court also overruled the district court's finding that voluntariness negates a claim of harassment, instead defining the test as whether Mr. Taylor's advances were "unwelcome," while acknowledging that determining unwelcomeness "presents difficult problems of proof."

HARRIS V. FORKLIFT SYSTEMS, INC., 510 U.S. 17 (1993)

Link to case: http://scholar.google.com/scholar_case?case=5109910086591041329

Question: For conduct to be actionable as "abusive work environment" harassment, must it seriously affect an employee's psychological well-being?

Answer: No.

Teresa Harris sued Forklift Systems, claiming that the conduct of the company's president, Charles Hardy, constituted "abusive work environment" harassment based on her gender in violation of Title VII of the Civil Rights Act of 1964. The magistrate found that Mr. Hardy made Ms. Harris the target of insults and sexual innuendoes in front of other employees. On several occasions Mr. Hardy asked Ms. Harris and other women to pick up objects he had thrown on the floor and get coins from his front pants pocket. Although the district court adopted the report of the magistrate and found that some of Mr. Hardy's conduct offended Ms. Harris and would be offensive to a reasonable woman, it ruled that it was not so severe as to affect her psychological well-being, nor did the court believe that Ms. Harris was subjectively so offended that she suffered injury. It thereby ruled that Ms. Harris had not been discriminated against under Title VII. After the U.S. Court of Appeals for the Sixth Circuit affirmed this ruling, the U.S. Supreme Court considered the case and reversed, stating succinctly, "Title VII comes into play before harassing conduct leads to a nervous breakdown." Further, "a discriminatorily abusive work environment, even one that does not seriously affect employees' psychological well-being, can and often will detract from the employee's job performance, discourage employees from remaining on the job, or keep them from advancing in their careers." The Court went on to reaffirm the *Meritor* standard that actionable conduct must create an "objectively hostile" work environment and must also be "subjectively" perceived by the victim as abusive.

ONCALE V. SUNDOWNER OFFSHORE SERVICES, INC., 523 U.S. 75 (1998)

Link to case: http://scholar.google.com/scholar_case?case=11566261664355830474

Question: Does abusive behavior between an employer and employee of the same sex qualify as discrimination under Title VII of the Civil Rights Act of 1964?

Answer: Yes.

Joseph Oncale worked in an eight-man crew on an oil rig in the Gulf of Mexico. On several occasions he was forcibly subjected to humiliating sex-related actions against him by some male coworkers in the presence of the rest of the crew and on one occasion was sexually assaulted by a male coworker who threatened him with rape. After complaints to supervisory personnel produced no remedial action, he quit, fearing he "would have been raped or forced to have sex." His discrimination suit in district court ended when the court granted summary judgment for the employer, finding that Title VII did not create a cause of action for harassment by same-sex coworkers, a ruling affirmed by the U.S. Court of Appeals for the Fifth Circuit. The U.S. Supreme Court reversed this decision, unanimously holding that workplace sexual harassment is actionable as sex discrimination under Title VII even if the harasser and the harassed are of the same sex. The Court relied on an earlier precedent in a case of racial discrimination that found that "because of the many facets of human motivation, it is unwise to presume as a matter of law that human beings of one definable group will not discriminate against other members of that group." The Court further held that the conduct "need not be motivated by sexual desire to support an inference of discrimination on the basis of sex." Instead, as already established in *Meritor* and *Harris*, the conduct must be so "objectively offensive" as to alter the "conditions" of the victim's employment.

CHAPTER 20

Sex

MERRILL ROTTER

ROY V. HARTOGS, 85 MISC. 2D 891 (1976)

Link to case: scholar.google.com/scholar_case?case=17414302291314969766

Question: Does sexual intercourse between psychiatrist and patient constitute malpractice?

Answer: Yes.

From 1969 to 1970, Dr. Renatus Hartogs treated Julie Roy, during which time he also engaged in sexual intercourse "as part of her prescribed therapy." Shortly thereafter, Ms. Roy sued Dr. Hartogs, alleging that she had been emotionally and mentally injured as a result of his improper treatment. Dr. Hartogs lost at trial and was found liable for both compensatory and punitive damages. On appeal, the court noted that the general right to sue for cases of seduction had been curtailed, but that this was a malpractice case, in which the doctor had failed to treat his patient within professionally acceptable standards. The court noted, however, that the trial jury had gone too far in assuming that Dr. Hartogs had neither the malicious intent nor level of recklessness necessary for punitive damages and that given Ms. Roy's long-standing psychiatric condition prior to the alleged malpractice, the award of $50,000 was excessive. The case was remanded for a new trial limited to compensatory damages up to $25,000. A concurring opinion cited Freud in noting that there is "common agreement of the harmful effects of sensual intimacies between patient and therapist."

CHAPTER 21

Questions on Tort Law

QUESTIONS

1. According to *Olmstead v. Zimring*, every state-hospitalized patient is entitled to timely community care once stable. Timely was defined as:
   A. Within 1 year.
   B. The Court did not give guidance on the amount of time.
   C. At a reasonable pace.
   D. Within 10 years.
   E. All deliberate speed.

2. A physician working with any health care third-party payer should:
   A. Understand and be prepared to appeal benefit claim denials if it is determined such denial could harm the patient
   B. Understand that the physician may still be liable for adverse treatment decisions
   C. Understand that there is a continued duty to treat the patient despite adverse benefit determinations by a third-party payer
   D. All of the above

3. In the United States, a plaintiff can recover damages for the negligent infliction of emotional distress based on:
   A. The impact rule
   B. The zone of danger
   C. Reasonable foreseeability
   D. Standards that vary from state to state
   E. Direct observation

4. ERISA stands for:
   A. Employee Retirement Income Security Act
   B. Employment Redress and Intervention Security Act
   C. Employees Right to Income and Security Act
   D. Employment Recovery and Income Stability Act

5. Which of the following is true about the role of sexual desire in cases of discrimination on the basis of sex?
   A. Sexual desire is a necessary element in determining the presence of discrimination.
   B. The victim's perception of the harasser's sexual desire is necessary.
   C. The conduct need not be motivated by sexual desire.
   D. Both the victim and the abuser must experience sexual desire.

6. A sexual relationship between a physician and a patient may be covered by malpractice insurance because:
   A. It is a side effect of psychotherapy.
   B. It is an occupational hazard for the psychotherapist.
   C. It is considered substandard clinical care.
   D. It is against the AMA ethical guidelines.
   E. It is against the APA ethical guidelines.

7. In *Hargrave v. Vermont*, Vermont Act 114, which allowed the state to override a durable power of attorney for a civilly committed individual, was found to violate Title II of the ADA because:
   A. The length of time that the individual had to be committed before the state could seek a court hearing for medication over objection was too short.
   B. Vermont Act 114 did not require a court order for medication over objection and thereby did not grant civilly committed individuals due process.
   C. There was no commensurate act allowing a person with physical illness to have his or her durable power of attorney overruled.
   D. Vermont Act 114 did not take into account emergency situations where medication over objection was needed to ensure the safety of people in the hospital.

8. How does an employee's response to sexual advances bear on a finding of sexual harassment?
   A. If she voluntarily participates, then she was not harassed.
   B. The response is not considered, only whether the advances were "unwelcome."
   C. An employee's repeated participation indicates it was acceptable.
   D. Acquiescence to sexual advances must be tied to an understanding that participation will result in advancement.
   E. All sexual contact between employees and supervisors qualifies as harassment.

9. The standards laid out regarding recovery for emotional harm in the case of *Thing v. La Chusa* (1989) state that the plaintiff must:
   A. Be a close relative, have witnessed the event, and have suffered emotional distress
   B. Have been in a position where he or she was at risk of harm, but not necessarily have suffered a physical impact
   C. Have been a direct victim rather than a bystander
   D. Have been partially responsible for the event him- or herself
   E. Have been a close relative of the defendant, mentally reconstructed the accident, and felt shock

10. "Reasonable foreseeability," as a policy regarding claims of negligent infliction of emotional damages, refers to:
    A. Whether the victim could have reasonably predicted the possibility of an accident, and therefore avoided it
    B. Whether a plaintiff could have reasonably seen a way to avoid the accident, and therefore shares liability due to contributory negligence
    C. Whether a defendant could have reasonably expected a negligent act to cause the resultant outcome, and therefore has a duty to the plaintiff
    D. Whether a judge could reasonably anticipate the outcome of a case, therefore resulting in a summary judgment
    E. Whether a lawyer could have reasonably calculated the amount of damages to be awarded, and therefore set his fee appropriately

11. According to *Mazza v. Medical Mutual Insurance Company of North Carolina*, punitive damages can be pursued from insurance companies for acts that are considered:
    A. Intentional
    B. Reckless
    C. Wanton
    D. Medical negligence
    E. All of the Above

12. The Americans with Disabilities Act was signed into law in what year?
    A. 1934
    B. 1964
    C. 1990
    D. 2008

13. James Carter, an employee of General Motors, sought workers' compensation benefits because:
    A. His hand was crushed by the machinery he operated on the assembly line.
    B. He witnessed someone get crushed by a forklift and could not longer come to work without experiencing disturbing flashbacks.
    C. He had a psychotic illness, and the symptoms were unremitting, thus making it impossible for him to return to work.
    D. The work Mr. Carter was asked to perform caused him emotional stress that led to psychosis.

14. You are the defendant in a case regarding a tort claim for emotional harm as a result of your alleged negligence. If you lose, what penalties could you face?
    A. The death penalty.
    B. Imprisonment.
    C. Corporal punishment.
    D. Monetary penalties.
    E. There is no penalty for emotional harm.

15. ERISA preemption regarding employee benefit plans means:
    A. The federal government is preempted from interfering with qualifying employee benefit plans.
    B. State laws are preempted insofar as they relate to the determination of benefits under an employee benefit plan, and the only remedies available are those given under the ERISA statute.
    C. Beneficiaries of ERISA plans are preempted from making claims against their plans.
    D. State and hospital surcharges are related to employee benefit plans and have to be preempted in order to standardize insurance rates.

16. A "hostile environment" violates Title VII of the Civil Rights Act of 1964 when it:
    A. Results in injury to the employee's physical health
    B. Results in injury to the employee's psychological health
    C. Alters the conditions of employment regardless of injury
    D. Enables the employer to exhibit frank hostility

17. Why did the U.S. Supreme Court overturn the appellate court decision in favor of Ms. Williams in her suit against Toyota?
    A. Wrist injuries are never serious enough to warrant protection under the ADA.
    B. The ADA does not protect against employment discrimination.
    C. Ms. Williams's impairment did not interfere with a "major life activity."
    D. Ms. Williams was found to be malingering.
    E. Ms. Williams had a factitious disorder.

18. An important factor in the *Wickline v. State* and *Wilson v. Blue Cross of Southern California* decisions was the physician's:
    A. Decision to appeal or not appeal a denied benefit claim
    B. Participation as an expert witness
    C. Credibility as a witness
    D. Membership on the applicable medical staff

19. *Dillon v. Legg* and *Thing v. La Chusa*, two cases involving requirements for seeking compensation regarding emotional harm, were decided for what jurisdiction?
    A. The State of New York
    B. The State of California
    C. Sacramento County
    D. The United States
    E. The United Nations

20. A defendant is responsible for negligently inflicting emotional harm only under certain circumstances. This is based on the concept of:
    A. Infinite liability
    B. Duty
    C. Malfeasance
    D. Tort
    E. Autonomy

21. Which of the following constitutes the test for an "objectively hostile" work environment?
    A. Descriptions available in peer-reviewed journals
    B. An expert's determination that the environment was hostile
    C. An environment that a "reasonable person" would find abusive or hostile
    D. The consensus of the workers in that environment

22. Employee benefit plans that provide health benefits to employees:
   A. Are rarely subject to ERISA provisions regarding benefits and claims for benefits
   B. Are subject to overlapping state and federal supervision
   C. May use prospective utilization review to deny treatment benefits even if recommended by a treating physician
   D. Have to pay additional hospital surcharges

23. For an incident to be covered by malpractice insurance, it:
   A. Must be an accident
   B. Must be intentional
   C. May never be intentional
   D. Depends on the details of the policy

24. In *Roy v. Hartogs*, the plaintiff was able to recover for her emotional harm because:
   A. Her psychiatrist was a registered sex offender.
   B. The sexual contact was nonconsensual.
   C. The behavior at issue constituted improper treatment.
   D. She had not given informed consent.
   E. Seduction often leads to psychological harm.

ANSWERS

1. **C**
   To satisfy the court ruling, the State of Georgia would have to maintain a list of people to be transferred that moved at a "reasonable pace." The rate "all deliberate speed" comes from the landmark *Brown v. Board of Education* decision concerning school desegregation.

2. **D**
   A physician should be prepared to appeal adverse benefit determinations of a patient's insurance or utilization reviewer if the physician believes that continued care is medically necessary. A physician still may be liable for failure to pursue an appeal and still may be liable in a state medical malpractice claim even if ERISA preempts any liability on the part of the third-party payer or reviewer. A physician generally has a duty to continue to treat a patient until the patient is stable and can be safely referred, even if continued benefits are denied.

3. **D**

    In the United States, each state has different criteria regarding a plaintiff's standing to sue for the negligent infliction of emotional distress. Some outdated standards include the impact rule (physical contact was required) and the zone of danger (an area in which a person was at risk of physical harm). A standard overturned in California but still used in some other jurisdictions is foreseeability (whether a defendant could have reasonably expected his actions to have had the resulting consequences). In *Thing v. La Chusa*, California adopted a set of standards that include whether the plaintiff is a close relative of the victim, directly observed the accident, and suffered emotional distress as a result.

4. **A**

    ERISA is the abbreviation for the Employee Retirement Income Security Act of 1974, which was passed by Congress to ensure federal uniformity of the regulation of employee benefits. When it was passed in 1974, health care benefits were provided on a fee-for-service basis, and managed care prospective review was not nearly as present as it later would become. The other choices are wrong for the obvious reasons.

5. **C**

    In *Oncale v. Sundowner Offshore Services*, the U.S. Supreme Court observed that although sexual harassment cases typically involve implicit or explicit proposals of sexual activity, the conduct "need not be motivated by sexual desire to support an inference of discrimination on the basis of sex." A trier of fact may, for instance, find discrimination when the harasser is motivated by general hostility toward the victim on the basis of her gender, even if the harasser and the victim are the same gender.

6. **C**

    Challenging emotional states and potential boundary violations are well-known risks of intensive psychotherapy for both therapists and patients. The AMA guidelines prohibit sexual relationships with active patients. The APA guidelines prohibit sexual relationships with both active and former patients. However, malpractice is not bound by any of these clinical or ethical standards. Malpractice ultimately is based on whether the clinical treatment fell below the accepted standard of care in the community.

7. **C**

    The central principle of the ruling in *Hargrave v. Vermont* is that Act 114 allowed for the overruling of the durable power of attorney for a mentally ill civilly committed individual but did not do so for a person with only physical illness. The length of time to seek a court order was 45 days, but this was not an issue in the court's decision (A). Act 114 did require a court order for medication over objection (B). The state hospital had the right to medicate over objection in emergency situations and therefore had nothing to do with Act 114 (D).

8. **B**

    In *Meritor Savings Bank v. Vinson*, the plaintiff participated in sexual activity with her supervisor multiple times over the course of 4 years. Although she stated that she did this out of fear of losing her job, the district court characterized her participation as "voluntary" because she did not resist and based the rejection of her claim in part on her willing participation. The U.S. Supreme Court ruled that voluntariness was not the central issue, instead defining the test as whether the advances were "unwelcome." Under this definition, not all sexual activity between an employee and a coworker or supervisor would qualify as harassment.

9. **A**

    In *Thing v. La Chusa*, the Supreme Court of California further defined the conditions that had been suggested in *Dillon v. Legg*. The court required that to have standing to seek damages for emotional harm, a plaintiff must be a close relative of the victim, have witnessed the event, and have suffered emotional distress. *Dillon v. Legg* had overturned *Amaya v. Home Ice, Fuel & Supply Co.* (1963), which stated that a plaintiff had to have been in a position where he or she was at actual risk of harm (the "zone of danger"). The legal reasoning in *Thing* included comments regarding the difficulty of determining whether a plaintiff was a direct victim or a bystander, and the case of *Molien v. Kaiser Foundation Hospitals* (1980) suggested that the *Dillon* guidelines did not apply to direct victims. *Dillon* also states that if the defendant is found not to be primarily liable due to the contributory negligence of the plaintiff, then that plaintiff cannot recover for emotional trauma. Option (E) is a combination of nonsensical propositions (that the plaintiff have been a close relative of the defendant); assertions from other cases (*Nazaroff v. Superior Court* [1978] asserted that liability could be extended if the plaintiff mentally reconstructed the event while the direct consequences were ongoing, but it was overturned by *Thing*); and older standards (the *Dillon* guideline of feeling shock as a direct result of the event eventually changed to the strict *Thing* criteria of emotional distress).

10. **C**

In the case of *Dillon v. Legg*, reasonable foreseeability refers to whether or not a defendant could have reasonably expected a negligent act to cause the resultant outcome. If so, then the negligent actor had a duty to the plaintiff. A victim's ability to avoid an accident does not obviate the duty of others to avoid acting in a negligent manner. *Dillon* states that if the defendant is found not to be primarily liable due to the contributory negligence of the plaintiff, then that plaintiff cannot recover for emotional trauma; however, that is not what is meant by reasonable foreseeability. The ability of a judge to anticipate the outcome of a case does not in itself allow him or her to make a summary judgment, and in any case it has nothing to do with the term in question. Lawyer's fees also bear no relation to the term.

11. **E**

In this case, the court was concerned with the issue of whether it was against public policy for an insurer to pay punitive damages for medical negligence of a physician under an insurance policy. The holding in the case illustrated that a policy may be construed to require the payment of punitive damages, and punitive damages may include not only intentional acts but also acts that are considered reckless or wanton. *Mazza v. Medical Mutual Insurance Company of North Carolina* makes clear that it is not, as a matter of law, against public policy for insurance contracts to cover these damages.

12. **C**

In 1934, the Communications Act was passed and called for affordable communications technology to be made available all people in the United States. Title IV of the ADA required that telecommunications options be made available for the disabled. The Civil Rights Act of 1964 made discrimination based on race, religion, gender, and national origin illegal. In 2008, President George W. Bush passed the ADA Amendments Act into law, further extending some of the protections of the original act, which was signed into law by President George H. W. Bush.

13. **D**

Someone does not need to suffer a physical injury on the job to receive workers' compensation (A). It does not need to be a single horrific event that causes the mental illness for someone to be able to receive workers' compensation but can actually just be mental illness due to the daily routine demands of the job as was the case with Mr. Carter (B). Mr. Carter's psychosis actually went into full remission (C). The

Michigan State Supreme Court ruled that Mr. Carter was not entitled to workers' compensation during periods of remission because at that point he was only predisposed to something that would interfere with his ability to work.

14. **D**

A tort claim is, by definition, governed by civil law. Capital punishment and imprisonment are possible penalties only under criminal law; corporal punishment, or the deliberate infliction of pain as a form of discipline, occurs mostly in the legal context of child abuse. Civil cases can result in fines or financial compensation and may also result in actions by organizations other than the court (such as official censures or the revocation of privileges). If emotional harm is proved, penalties are certainly possible.

15. **B**

Section 514 of the ERISA statute preempts any state law that relates to employee benefit plans. As such, traditional state tort claims such as negligence and breach of contract are not available against the employee benefit plan because of Section 514. There are very narrow and small exceptions that case law has carved out, but ultimately ERISA greatly restricts the ability of employee plan participants to sue their plans for adverse benefit determinations. The federal government is not preempted from regulating plans, nor are plan beneficiaries preempted from suing them. The last option relates to the *New York State Conference of Blue Cross and Blue Shield Plans et al. v. Travelers Insurance Co. et al* case, but the finding in that case was that surcharges are not related to the administration of the employee benefit plans and so therefore are not preempted.

16. **C**

In both *Meritor Savings Bank v. Vinson* and *Harris v. Forklift Systems, Inc.*, the U.S. Supreme Court stated that a "hostile environment" exists when discrimination is "sufficiently severe and pervasive" so as to alter the conditions of employment. In many instances plaintiffs claim that the hostile environment resulted in injury to their physical or psychological health, and experts are asked to opine regarding the extent of those damages. But the Supreme Court ruled in *Harris* that "Title VII comes into play before harassing conduct leads to a nervous breakdown." In other words, the existence of a hostile environment alone is sufficient to qualify as discrimination regardless of whether the plaintiff experienced additional injury to physical or psychological well-being.

17. **C**

Despite having carpal tunnel syndrome, Ms. Williams retained the ability to perform most activities of daily living. It appeared as though her only limitation was being able to continue working as a manual laborer. There is no class of injury or illness that is not open to ADA protection; it depends on the effects of the condition (A). Title I of the ADA specifically prohibits discrimination in employment on the basis of disability (B). There is nothing to suggest Ms. Williams was malingering or that her carpal tunnel syndrome was factitious (D, E).

18. **A**

The *Wickline* and *Wilson* decisions involved fact patterns where the physician did not appeal an insurance adverse benefit determination. This fact was more dispositive for the underlying issue in the *Wickline* case than in the *Wilson* case, but both cases illustrate the role of the physician's final decision. The court held in *Wilson* that the physician's failure to place an appeal did not relieve the third-party reviewer of the potential for liability.

19. **B**

Though the legal reasoning described in the opinions has served as the basis for many other state policies, the landmark cases regarding negligent infliction of emotional damages were decided by the Supreme Court of California and therefore apply only to the state of California. *Dillon v. Legg* initially started in the county of Sacramento, but the legal precedent was set for the entire state. New York has a separate legal system, though it has been informed by the debate surrounding the decisions of other states. The U.S. Supreme Court has not set a policy for the entire country to follow, and the United Nations is an international organization consisting of nearly 200 countries.

20. **B**

Duty is a concept referring to a legal obligation and only exists between two parties under specifically defined circumstances. Infinite liability (the potential for anyone to sue for damages stemming from any particular negligent act) is a problem that the courts attempt to avoid by placing restrictions on who has legal standing to bring a lawsuit. Malfeasance is an intentional wrongful act, often in an official context. Tort also means an injury or wrongful act, but it may be intentional or accidental. Autonomy is an unrelated concept regarding the ability of rational people to make informed decisions for themselves.

21. **C**

In determining whether a work environment is "objectively hostile," the fact-finder must consider how a "reasonable person" would react under similar circumstances. In *Harris v. Forklift Systems, Inc.*, the U.S. Supreme Court cited several elements that might be used to define such an environment, including discriminatory intimidation, ridicule, and insult, as well as the environment's impact on an employee's performance, desire to advance, and motivation to stay on the job. Despite these signposts, the determination rests on the "reasonable person." Attorneys for both plaintiffs and defendants often attempt to introduce expert testimony to define this standard, but courts are likely to limit the role an expert can play in defining the reactions of a "reasonable person," leaving this up to the jury.

22. **D**

The purpose of ERISA is to regulate employee benefit plans that companies set up for their employees. Health care benefits are often part of these benefits. To control costs, these companies often will use prospective utilization review companies to determine whether to allow or deny benefits under the terms of the plan. These benefit determinations are subject to ERISA's specific provisions and remedies. If any state law "relates" to an employee benefit plan, it is preempted so there is no overlapping state regulation.

23. **D**

Cases of negligence are ones in which the harm caused was not intended. However, that is different from whether or not the action itself was intentional as opposed to an accident. In *Aetna v. McCabe*, the court noted that, in general, behavior can be considered malpractice whether it was accidental or intentional, but in this case the critical fact was that Dr. McCabe's policy did not specifically exclude intentional actions from coverage.

24. **C**

This case was treated as a pure malpractice case in which the sexual contact between psychiatrist and patient was deemed improper and below accepted professional standards. Dr. Hartogs was not a sexual offender, and their was no allegation that the patient had been coerced or uninformed. The court noted that the right to recover a sum of money for seduction as a general matter had been abolished, but that this case was one of malpractice, not seduction per se.

SECTION V

Criminal Law and Incarceration

This section describes cases that involve defendants at various levels of the criminal justice system. The chapters are divided between cases that cover procedural issues such as competencies to confess and stand trial and substantive issues, including the standards for guilt in substance abuse cases, diminished capacity, and legal insanity. As a rule, the U.S. Constitution leaves criminal law procedures to the states. These cases, therefore, often reflect the U.S. Supreme Court's judgment as to the minimum standards required by the Constitution; great variability among state jurisdictions still remains. These cases contain important reflections on the mind, mental illness, psychiatric treatment, and the balancing of individual rights and state power.

Two additional chapters included herein review the rights of prisoners and the death penalty. For forensic practitioners and administrators in correctional institutions, familiarity with the standard of care required, at the very least, by the Constitution is critically important. The death penalty cases provide a unique window into the continually changing view of mental disability, development, and personhood. Most of the cases involve an individual who is appealing a death sentence that he or she believes violates the Eighth Amendment prohibiting cruel and unusual punishment, with an emphasis on the mental age and/or mental functioning that should be an exception to such a sentence. Not surprisingly, the American Psychiatric Association has written forceful briefs in nearly all these cases.

CHAPTER 22

Criminal Procedure

MICHAEL GREENSPAN, AMAR MEHTA, AND
MERRILL ROTTER

MIRANDA V. ARIZONA, 384 U.S. 436 (1966)

Link to case: http://caselaw.lp.findlaw.com/scripts/getcase.pl?navby=case&court=us&vol=384&page=436

Question: Are police required to inform a suspect of his or her rights to remain silent and to have an attorney present?

Answer: Yes.

In 1963, Ernesto Miranda was arrested for kidnapping and rape. At trial, his attorney objected to the admission of his confession, contending that it was not voluntary. The objection was overruled, and Mr. Miranda was convicted. Upon arrest, Mr. Miranda had signed a confession that included a statement as to its voluntariness and with "full knowledge of my legal rights." However, he had not been explicitly advised by the police of his right to counsel or his right to remain silent. The Arizona Supreme Court upheld the conviction, and Mr. Miranda appealed to the U.S. Supreme Court, asserting that his Fifth and Sixth Amendment rights had been violated. The Court ruled that due to the inherently coercive nature of custodial interrogation, a suspect must be "clearly informed" of his rights and must waive them.

NORTH CAROLINA V. ALFORD, 400 U.S. 25 (1970)

Link to case: http://scholar.google.com/scholar_case?case=14055791673999770436

Question: Can a defendant plead guilty even though he maintains his innocence?

Answer: Yes.

In 1963, Henry Alford was indicted with first-degree murder, a charge carrying a potential death penalty in North Carolina. Faced with strong evidence of guilt, along with state procedure that allowed for a mitigation of punishment to life imprisonment with a guilty plea (as opposed to a jury conviction), Mr. Alford entered a guilty plea. On the stand, Mr. Alford stated that he was entering his plea only to avoid the death penalty, saying, "I'm not guilty but I plead guilty." Following his plea, while incarcerated, Mr. Alford sought postconviction relief (first at the state level and later in the federal court of appeals) and failed in several jurisdictions, wherein his plea was felt to be a "voluntary and intelligent choice." In 1967, the Fourth Circuit Court of Appeals reversed the guilty plea, finding it to be involuntary because its principal motivation was fear of the death penalty. In a 6–3 holding, The U.S. Supreme Court reversed this decision. Despite Mr. Alford's claim of innocence, the Court felt that (1) the strong evidence supporting his guilt and (2) his representation by competent counsel resulted in a valid guilty plea. The fear of the death penalty, in and of itself, is not adequately coercive to invalidate a guilty plea within the meaning of the Fifth Amendment.

COLORADO V. CONNELLY, 479 U.S. 157 (1986)

Link to case: http://scholar.google.com/scholar_case?case=13661442250005953902

Question: Is coercive police activity required for a finding of lack of voluntariness of a confession?

Answer: Yes

On August 18, 1983, Francis Connelly approached a police officer in Denver, Colorado, and stated that he had committed a murder and wanted to confess. The police officer provided a Miranda warning and later stated that he did not believe Mr. Connelly to be clearly under the influence of substances or mentally ill at the time of the confession. The next morning, however, when questioned by the public defender, Mr. Connelly appeared confused and stated that he had confessed as a result of auditory hallucinations. Following restoration for lack of competence to stand trial, the Colorado trial court suppressed the confession, finding that it was not the product of a defendant's "rational intellect and free will" (citing *Townsend v. Sain* [1963], an earlier U.S. Supreme Court decision). The Colorado Supreme Court affirmed this on initial appeal. In a 7–2 holding, the U.S. Supreme Court reversed the decision, holding that coercive police activity is *required* to allow the suppression of a confession based on violation of the Due Process Clause of the Fourteenth Amendment. The Court allowed that mental illness is relevant to a defendant's susceptibility to state coercion, but that such illness alone and its effect on "voluntariness" do not constitute a due process violation.

ROBINSON V. CALIFORNIA, 370 U.S. 660 (1962)

Link to case: http://caselaw.lp.findlaw.com/scripts/getcase.pl?navby=case&court=us&vol=370&page=660

Question: Is the status of drug addiction a crime?

Answer: No.

A California statute in 1962 made it a misdemeanor crime to "be addicted to the use of narcotics," further defined at trial as "a status or condition and not an act." Police officers in Los Angeles stopped Lawrence Robinson and observed track marks on his arms that they believed to be from intravenous drug abuse (Mr. Robinson claimed they were the result of an allergic condition). He was not intoxicated or withdrawing at the time and was not acting in a disruptive or antisocial manner. He was found guilty, and the verdict was affirmed on appeal. The case was then appealed to the U.S. Supreme Court for inflicting a "cruel and unusual punishment" in violation of the Eighth Amendment as applicable to the states through the Fourteenth Amendment. The Court noted that a brief imprisonment in itself was neither cruel nor unusual, but "[e]ven one day in prison would be a cruel and unusual punishment for the 'crime' of having a common cold." It was also noted that addiction could even occur "innocently or involuntarily," such as by exposure in utero or starting with a legitimate prescription. The statute was found unconstitutional, and the decision was reversed.

POWELL V. TEXAS, 392 U.S. 514 (1968)

Link to case: http://caselaw.lp.findlaw.com/scripts/getcase.pl?navby=case&court=us&vol=392&page=514

Question: Is public intoxication a crime if it is a result of alcoholism?

Answer: Yes.

A Texas statute in 1968 made it a crime, punishable by a fine, to "be found in a state of intoxication in a public place." Leroy Powell was arrested and found guilty of public intoxication in Austin and appealed to a county court. He argued that chronic alcoholism was a disease, and to criminally punish someone for suffering from a disease would be "cruel and unusual punishment" in violation of the Eighth Amendment, as applicable to the states through the Fourteenth Amendment (as decided in *Robinson v. California*). A new trial was held, and Mr. Powell was again found guilty. When he appealed to the U.S. Supreme Court, the resulting opinion included a review of the "disease" concept of alcoholism, as well as the "substantial disagreement within the medical profession" regarding its definitions and limitations. Medical testimony noted that "these individuals have a compulsion ... while not completely overpowering, [it is] an exceedingly strong influence," and the Court decided that there was not enough clarity to remove responsibility. The guilty verdict was upheld on the grounds that Mr. Powell was not convicted for the status of being an alcoholic but rather for the act of being intoxicated in public at a specific time.

CHAPTER 23

Criminal Competencies

MATTHEW W. GROVER

DUSKY V. U.S. 362 U.S. 402 (1960)

Link to case: http://scholar.google.com/scholar_case?case=2877494138671044176

Question: Is basic knowledge about one's charges enough to be competent to stand trial?

Answer: No.

Milton Dusky was a 33-year-old man diagnosed with schizophrenia when he was charged, along with two juvenile codefendants, of abducting and raping a teenage girl. His attorney raised the issue of his competence to stand trial, and Mr. Dusky was hospitalized for 4 months at a federal hospital for examination. The competency report noted that he was not able to understand the legal proceedings against him, nor could he assist counsel. One expert testified that he had difficulty with reality testing and was suspicious. The trial judge in the U.S. District Court in Missouri found him competent to stand trial, noting that he was oriented to time and place, had some recollection of events, and appeared to be able to assist counsel. Mr. Dusky was convicted and sentenced to 45 years. The U.S. Court of Appeals, Eighth Circuit, affirmed his conviction. The U.S. Supreme Court reversed and held that the record did not sufficiently support the finding of competency to stand trial. While Mr. Dusky understood the basic elements of the court proceedings and the charges, he was unable to assist counsel due to his psychosis. The court held that the test of a defendant's competency to stand trial is "whether he has sufficient present ability to consult with his lawyer with a reasonable degree of rational understanding - and whether he has a rational as well as factual understanding of the proceedings against him."

WILSON V. U.S. 391 F.2D 460 (1968)

Link to case: http://openjurist.org/391/f2d/460/wilson-v-united-states

Question: Must permanent retrograde amnesia render a defendant incompetent to stand trial?

Answer: No.

On October 2, 1964, Robert Wilson and his partner carjacked a man at gunpoint and robbed a pharmacy. As a result of the ensuing high-speed chase with a police cruiser, the defendants crashed the car into a tree. The partner died, but Mr. Wilson, who fractured his skull and was unconscious for 3 weeks, survived. Upon regaining consciousness, Mr. Wilson had retrograde amnesia and was unable to recall the circumstances surrounding the incident. He was initially found incompetent to stand trial due to his retrograde amnesia, and a district court judge had him committed to St. Elizabeth's Hospital in Washington, DC, for 14 months. In November 1966, he was found competent to stand trial and convicted. On appeal, Mr. Wilson raised the question as to whether "it is a denial of due process [fair trial per the Fifth Amendment] or of the right to effective assistance of counsel [Sixth Amendment] to try a defendant suffering from such a loss of memory." The U.S. Court of Appeals, District of Columbia Circuit, found that a loss of memory in this instance did not make the defendant incompetent as long as he had the ability to extrinsically construct a knowledge of what happened, follow the proceedings against him, discuss the proceedings rationally with his attorney, and testify on his own behalf. These rules applied as long as the availability of other evidence made the defendant's personal memory less critical to his defense. The case was remanded for consideration of the above.

JACKSON V. INDIANA, 406 U.S. 715 (1972)

Link to case: http://scholar.google.com/scholar_case?case=3353749416334368664

Question: Can a defendant be committed indefinitely if he is found incompetent to stand trial?

Answer: No.

In 1968, Theon Jackson was charged in Marion, Indiana, with two counts of robbery of two women whose stolen items were valued at nine dollars. A competency evaluation was ordered, as he was described as a "deaf mute" who was unable to read and write and who communicated only through limited sign language. He was found incompetent to stand trial, and both examiners found it unlikely that he would improve over the long term. He was committed to the Indiana Department of Mental Health until the department could certify that Mr. Jackson was "sane." Mr. Jackson's counsel filed a motion for a new trial, contending that there was no evidence that his client was "insane," nor was there evidence that he would ever be restored to competence for the purposes of standing trial. His counsel argued that the commitment amounted to a "life sentence" without a conviction and therefore deprived Mr. Jackson of his rights to due process and equal protection under the Fourteenth Amendment and violated the Eighth Amendment prohibition against cruel and unusual punishment. The trial court denied his motion, and the Supreme Court of Indiana affirmed the denial. The U.S. Supreme Court reversed and agreed with Mr. Jackson's argument. The court also stated that indefinite commitment as a result of incompetency violated due process and that an incompetent defendant cannot be held more than what is considered a reasonable period of time to determine "whether there is a substantial probability that he will attain that capacity in the foreseeable future." If capacity restoration is unlikely, civil commitment proceedings would be required to justify further confinement.

DROPE V. MISSOURI, 420 U.S. 162 (1975)

Link to case: http://scholar.google.com/scholar_case?case=12110713099598535891

Question: Should a judge interrupt criminal proceedings if a defendant appears to be incompetent?

Answer: Yes.

In February 1969, James Drope was indicted with two other men on charges of raping his wife. His counsel filed a motion for continuance in order for Mr. Drope to be examined and receive psychiatric treatment. When this motion was initially rejected, counsel expressed that Mr. Drope was not of sound mind and requested further psychiatric evaluation before the case went to trial. His objection was denied, and the case proceeded forward. After his wife's testimony on the first day of the trial, during which she noted his bizarre behavior and an attempt to choke her on the preceding day, Mr. Drope shot himself in the abdomen. When he failed to show up to court the next morning, his counsel moved for a mistrial, which was denied. Mr. Drope was convicted and sentenced to life in prison. Mr. Drope's counsel filed a motion for a new trial, which was denied. In 1971, Mr. Drope filed a motion to vacate his judgment and conviction based upon a violation of his constitutional rights. This motion was again denied. On appeal to the U.S. Supreme Court, the Court concluded that the record revealed a failure to give proper weight to the information that came to light at the trial suggesting Mr. Drope's incompetence. In addition, it noted that the Court should reconsider competence at any point in a trial where circumstances suggest a change that would render the accused unable to meet the standards of competency to stand trial. In Mr. Drope's case, there was sufficient evidence to question his competency, and the correct course was to suspend the trial until competency evaluation could be completed. The conviction and sentence were reversed, and the case was remanded. The Court also noted that the state was free to retry Mr. Drope, assuming that he was competent to be tried.

GODINEZ V. MORAN, 509 U.S. 389 (1993)

Link to case: http://scholar.google.com/scholar_case?case=13448720628873766473

Question: Is the standard to waive constitutional rights higher than the standard for competency to stand trial?

Answer: No.

Richard Moran entered the Red Pearl Saloon in Las Vegas, Nevada, on August 2, 1984, and shot and killed the bartender and a bar patron before removing the cash register. Nine days later, he shot and killed his former wife before shooting himself in the abdomen and slitting his wrists. Mr. Moran survived, and on August 13, he confessed to the killings. After pleading not guilty to three counts of first-degree murder, he was found competent to stand trial by two psychiatrists. Mr. Moran subsequently informed the court that he wished to dismiss his attorneys and change his plea to guilty. The court accepted his waiver of counsel and his guilty pleas. A three-judge court sentenced him to death on January 21, 1985. In 1987, he sought postconviction relief in the state court on grounds that he was incompetent to represent himself, but the trial court and the Supreme Court of Nevada rejected this claim. He subsequently filed a writ of habeas corpus petition in the U.S. District Court of Nevada, which was denied. The Ninth Circuit reversed, concluding that the Due Process Clause of the Fourteenth Amendment required the court to hold a hearing with regard to Mr. Moran's competency before accepting his dismissal of counsel and change of plea. The Ninth Circuit specifically stated that that competency to waive constitutional rights required a higher level of mental functioning, which it termed a "reasoned choice" standard. The U.S. Supreme Court reversed, rejecting the notion that competency in matters of pleading guilty or waiving right counsel was to be measured by a higher standard than the one outlined in *Dusky v. U.S.*

COOPER V. OKLAHOMA, 517 U.S. 348 (1996)

Link to case: http://scholar.google.com/scholar_case?case=2215296136817695478

Question: Is preponderance of the evidence the appropriate standard for determining competency to stand trial?

Answer: Yes.

Mr. Cooper was charged in the murder of an 86-year-old man in 1989. A jury found him guilty of first-degree murder, and the court concurred with the jury's recommendation of the death penalty. On five separate occasions before and during the trial, Mr. Cooper's competence was called into question. His behavior over the course of the trial included refusing to change out of his prison garb because he believed the clothes were "burning" him, talking to himself and an imaginary "spirit" who provided him counsel, and expressing a fear that his counsel wanted to kill him. Mr. Cooper's attorney moved for a mistrial or additional investigation into his competence but was denied. The Court of Criminal Appeals rejected the argument that Oklahoma's presumption of competence and statutory requirement that incompetence be established by clear and convincing evidence violated his due process. The U.S. Supreme Court reversed on appeal, finding that the heightened standard of clear and convincing evidence was not protective of the defendant's rights under the Due Process Clause of the Fourteenth Amendment because it "imposes a significant risk of erroneous determination" that an incompetent defendant is found competent. The result of such a determination threatens the "basic fairness of the trial itself," and the defendant's right to be tried while competent outweighs the state's interest in operating an efficient criminal justice system. The standard of proof must be preponderance of the evidence.

INDIANA V. EDWARDS, 128 S. CT. 2379 (2008)

Link to case: http://scholar.google.com/scholar_case?case=15676731200684587378

Question: Are there different standards for competency to stand trial and competency to represent oneself?

Answer: Yes.

Ahmad Edwards, a man with schizophrenia, attempted to steal a pair of shoes from the Parisian Department Store in Indianapolis in July 1999. After being discovered, he fired a gun at a store security guard, injuring a bystander. Mr. Edwards fled and was apprehended by an FBI agent, who shot him in the thigh after Mr. Edwards refused to drop his weapon. He was charged with attempted murder. Mr. Edwards's competency to stand trial was questioned several times, and he required restoration of his fitness on two occasions. He was convicted of all charges and appealed to the intermediate appellate court in Indiana, arguing that the refusal to permit him to represent himself denied him his constitutional right of self-representation. The court agreed and ordered a new trial. The Indiana Supreme Court affirmed the intermediate appellate court's decision, finding that Mr. Edwards's Sixth Amendment right to self-representation had been violated. The U.S. Supreme Court vacated the judgment of the Supreme Court of Indiana and remanded the case for further proceedings, stating that the standard outlined in *Dusky* applied to those with counsel. The standard for competency to stand trial was not the standard to determine competency for defendants to conduct trial proceedings by themselves. Therefore, the U.S. Constitution permits states to insist upon representation by counsel for those incompetent to conduct trial proceedings by themselves but competent to stand trial under *Dusky*.

CHAPTER 24

Diminished Capacity

MICHAEL GREENSPAN

PEOPLE V. PATTERSON, 39 N.Y.2D 288 (1976)

Link to case: http://scholar.google.com/scholar_case?case=6754859816004446983

Question: Is it constitutional in New York to place the burden of proof for extreme emotional disturbance (EED) on the defendant?

Answer: Yes

Gordon Patterson had an unstable and abusive relationship with his wife. In December 1970, Mr. Patterson observed his wife scantily dressed with John Northrup, her paramour. Mr. Patterson shot Mr. Northrup twice in the head at close range. At trial, Mr. Patterson claimed both that the gun had gone off accidentally and that he had been acting in a state of extreme emotional disturbance. Under the New York statute, EED could potentially mitigate a murder conviction to manslaughter. The burden of proving EED was placed on the defendant. At trial, Mr. Patterson was found guilty of murder. He unsuccessfully appealed, based on the primary contention that his due process right under the Fourteenth Amendment had been violated because the jury had been instructed that the defense bore the burden to prove EED. The New York Court of Appeals affirmed the decision against Mr. Patterson, holding that the New York EED law did not negate the "fundamental" constitutional principle that the state must prove all the elements of a crime. Placing the burden of proving EED on the defense, as defined in the New York statutory scheme, does not violate due process protection.

IBN-TAMAS V. U.S. 407 A.2D 626 (1979)

Link to case: http://scholar.google.com/ scholar_case?case=8618054616035755185

Question: Should testimony about a recognized syndrome in a defendant be excluded from evidence because of its potential prejudicial impact on the jury?

Answer: No.

Beverly Ibn-Tamas was convicted of second-degree murder in the Superior Court of Washington, DC. Ms. Ibn-Tamas had shot her husband after years of physical abuse at his hands. On the morning of the incident, her husband had assaulted her, pointed a gun at her head, and told her to leave the family's residence or suffer severe retribution. At trial, the defense attempted to enter testimony of Dr. Lenore Walker, a clinical psychologist. Dr. Walker discussed the "battered woman syndrome." She opined that the defendant did, in fact, suffer from said syndrome and therefore was acting in what in her mind was self-defense. The trial court did not allow entry of this evidence, feeling that it would infringe on the province of the jury to assess the credibility of witnesses and that it presupposed that her husband was, in fact, a batterer. The DC Court of Appeals reversed the decision, stating that the testimony should not have been excluded. It reasoned that the expert was providing important background information that was "beyond the ken" of an ordinary jury. Therefore, the probative value of the information outweighed any potential prejudicial effect. The case was remanded for further consideration, including the now admissible testimony.

PEOPLE V. SAILLE, 54 CAL. 3D 1103 (1991)

Link to case: http://scholar.google.com/scholar_case? case=10687954333870937195

Issue: Can voluntary intoxication be used to reduce a murder charge to manslaughter in California?

Answer: No.

Manuel De Jesus Saille became severely drunk at a local bar, Eva's Café, in California. Upon being "turned down" twice for more alcohol, Mr. Saille left the bar after threatening to return and kill the bartender. He returned with a firearm. In the struggle that ensued with the bar's security, a bystander was shot and killed. Mr. Saille's blood alcohol level several hours after the shooting was 0.14. Mr. Saille was found guilty of murder at trial and appealed based on the contention that the jury instruction that voluntary intoxication was only relevant to "specific intent to kill" was inadequate. The court of appeals, and ultimately the California Supreme Court, affirmed the trial court's guilty finding. The court opined that the state's new penal law had limited voluntary intoxication as a defense to cases only where there was evidence that it affected a defendant's ability to form specific intent, in this case, a premeditated decision to kill another person. Voluntary intoxication, alone, could not be a reason for reducing the crime to manslaughter.

MONTANA V. EGELHOFF, 518 U.S. 37 (1996)

Link to case: http://scholar.google.com/scholar_case?case=2969282020576743127

Question: Does the Montana law excluding evidence about voluntary intoxication as related to mental state in a criminal offense violate due process?

Answer: No.

In July 1992, James Egelhoff met Roberta Pavola and John Christenson while camping in Montana. The group picked mushrooms and soon engaged in a night of binge drinking. At around midnight, police officers discovered Mr. Egelhoff in the back of the car, shouting obscenities and with a blood alcohol level of 0.36. Ms. Pavola and Mr. Christenson lay dead in the car, each with a single gunshot wound to the head. Mr. Egelhoff had gun residue on his hands, and the weapon of the crime lay on the floor of the parked car. The Montana statute of murder required that the defendant "purposely" or "knowingly" engaged in the murderous act. The trial jury was instructed not to consider the defendant's drunkenness at the time of the crime and ultimately found Egelhoff guilty. The Montana Supreme Court reversed the guilty finding, reasoning that the due process protections under the Fourteenth Amendment require that all relevant evidence, including that of voluntary intoxication, be considered. On certiorari, the U.S. Supreme Court reversed the appeal, agreeing with the trial court's suppression of this mental state evidence. The Court relied on historical and common law arguments to hold that the exclusion of voluntary intoxication in violent crimes was not a violation of due process.

CHAPTER 25

Insanity

KATYA FRISCHER

M'NAGHTEN'S CASE, 8 ENG. REP. 718 (1843)

Link to case: http://www.stanford.edu/group/psylawseminar/M%27Naghten.htm

Question: Can a defendant be found not guilty by reason of insanity (NGRI) in a criminal case if, as a result of mental illness, he cognitively did not know what he was doing or that it was wrong?

Answer: Yes.

On January 20, 1843, Mr. M'Naghten shot British prime minister Robert Peel's secretary, Mr. Drummond, while attempting to shoot Mr. Peel. Mr. Drummond died from his wounds. M'Naghten was found NGRI by the jury. Evidence presented in court indicated Mr. M'Naghten was mentally ill with persecutory delusions, which resulted in his inability to control his behavior at the time of the crime. Due to public outrage, Queen Victoria appealed to the judges in the House of Lords to answer general questions about the standard for legal insanity (e.g., What is the law regarding a defendant's guilt if he is afflicted with delusions but knows he is acting contrary to the law? Can a physician testify as to the state of mind of a defendant if he did not examine him prior to trial?). The judges opined that in order to be adjudicated not guilty by reason of insanity the defendant has to be mentally ill to the extent that he is incapable of knowing what he is doing or, if he knows what he is doing, that he knows that what he is doing is wrong. This cognitive, knowledge of right and wrong criterion has come to be known as the M'Naghten standard.

DURHAM V. U.S. 214 F.2D 862 (1954)

Link to case: http://scholar.google.com/scholar_case?case=1244686235948852364

Question: Is the *M'Naghten* "right/wrong" standard outdated, and should a more "modern" criterion be whether or not the criminal actions were the product of a mental disease or defect?

Answer: Yes.

In 1954 the U.S. Court of Appeals, District of Columbia Circuit, reviewed the trial court's housebreaking conviction of Monte Durham. Mr. Durham had a well-documented history of mental illness since the age of 17. He was reported to have hallucinations and had been hospitalized several times at St. Elizabeth's Psychiatric Hospital. He had been variably diagnosed with "psychosis with psychopathic personality" as well as "without mental disorder, psychopathic personality." The court of appeals reversed Mr. Durham's conviction on two grounds: (1) the trial court erred in stating that there was "no" evidence of mental disorder, when there was "some" evidence, shifting the burden to the state to prove sanity as per the existing insanity defense standard; and (2) in light of more modern conceptions of mental processes, the standard for legal insanity should be changed to "product of mental disease or defect" from the existing *M'Naghten* right/wrong test and/or irresistible impulse. This was known as the *Durham*, or product, rule.

WASHINGTON V. U.S., 390 F.2D 444 (1967)

Link to case: http://scholar.google.com/scholar_case?case=11121900497855531360

Question: Should an expert witness be allowed to testify to the ultimate question in an insanity defense case?

Answer: No.

Thomas Washington was convicted by jury of rape, robbery, and assault with a deadly weapon in Washington, DC, following an unsuccessful insanity defense. During the trial there was a wide range of testimony by psychiatric experts on both sides regarding the mental health of the defendant. Mr. Washington appealed the conviction to the U.S. Court of Appeals for the DC Circuit. The court found that the psychiatric evidence presented at trial was "more confusing than clarifying," at times omitted important evidence, and was an "abstract mass of philosophical discussion." However, it reasoned that although much of the information presented to the jury may have been conclusory, full of medical jargon, and confusing, the jury ultimately got enough facts to be able to make a decision regarding the defendant's mental illness and culpability. The court, in an opinion by Justice David Bazelon, ruled that the jury, not the psychiatric experts, should decide to what extent the alleged offense was a *product* of mental illness. The court advised that the trial judge should give explanatory instructions in open court regarding the proper role of the expert and the jury.

FRENDAK V. U.S., 408 A.2D 364 (1979)

Link to case: http://scholar.google.com/scholar_case?case=8884757738165900061

Question: Can a defendant with mental illness whose sanity at the time of the crime is in question competently refuse to raise an insanity defense?

Answer: Yes.

Paula Frendak was convicted of first-degree homicide in Washington, DC, in 1974 for killing a coworker, Willard Titlow, and carrying a pistol without a license. After the shooting, Ms. Frendak left Washington and traveled abroad until she was extradited to Washington from Abu Dhabi. She had a history of mental illness, including a history of hallucinations and delusions. She had several competency hearings and was found competent to stand trial on the fourth evaluation. After her conviction, she appealed, stating that the trial judge inappropriately raised the insanity defense over her competent objections. The DC Court of Appeals enumerated several good reasons to refuse the insanity defense and ruled that if a defendant has acted intelligently and voluntarily, a trial court must defer to his or her decision to waive the insanity defense. However, the trial court should have the ability to raise the defense if a defendant is not capable of making or has not made an intelligent and voluntary decision. A finding of competency to stand trial does not imply competence to make decisions about the insanity defense. The case was remanded to clarify if the defendant was capable of intelligently refusing the insanity defense.

JONES V. U.S., 463 U.S. 354 (1983)

Link to case: http://scholar.google.com/scholar_case?case=5221664652529148549

Question: Can an insanity acquittee be confined longer than he would have been had he been found guilty of the same crime?

Answer: Yes.

Michael Jones was arrested for attempting to steal a jacket from a department store in the District of Columbia. He was charged with misdemeanor petty larceny and eventually found not guilty by reason of insanity. He was committed at St. Elizabeth's Hospital with a diagnosis of schizophrenia. At a court hearing he requested to be released or recommitted under a civil commitment statute, stating that he had been hospitalized for longer than the period he would have spent in prison if he had been convicted. He was denied and appealed to the DC Court of Appeals on the grounds that his Fourteenth Amendment right to due process had been violated. The appellate court, after several hearings, affirmed the trial court finding. The U.S. Supreme Court heard the case and ruled that a finding of insanity at trial is sufficient to justify commitment at a preponderance of the evidence standard (lower than the civil commitment clear and convincing requirement), since the verdict was based on a finding of mental illness and a criminal act, which is by definition, dangerousness. Furthermore, commitment as an insanity acquittee serves a different purpose than incarceration, and there is no necessary correlation between the severity of the offense and the length of time necessary for recovery. Insanity acquittees constitute a special class and can be treated differently from civil patients.

U.S. V. TORNIERO, 735 F.2D 725 (2D CIR. CONN. 1984)

Link to case: http://scholar.google.com/scholar_case?case=11490969042080455149

Question: Is an individual with compulsive gambling necessarily legally insane with respect to all behaviors that may be associated with his gambling behavior?

Answer: No.

John Torniero, a jewelry store manager, was indicted for interstate transportation of jewelry worth $750,000 stolen from his employer. He argued that a compulsion to gamble rendered him legally insane. After extensive testimony by psychiatrists, the trial court ruled that the relationship between gambling and the urge to steal is tenuous and was irrelevant to the issue of insanity. Mr. Torniero was convicted and then appealed to the U.S. Court of Appeals for the Second Circuit, stating that the trial judge erred by refusing to present the evidence about compulsive gambling to the jury. The court of appeals affirmed, explaining that under the American Law Institute (ALI) test a person is not responsible for criminal conduct if at the time of such conduct as a result of mental disease or defect he lacks substantial capacity either to appreciate the wrongfulness of his conduct or to conform his conduct to the requirements of the law. In this case the evidence would be relevant if the defendant could prove that compulsive gambling is a mental disease or defect capable of making him unable to resist the urge to steal. The court reasoned that in order for it to consider psychiatric evidence for the purposes of insanity, there should be substantial acceptance in the discipline that compulsive gambling is a mental illness and that there is a nexus between gambling and stealing. It found that the trial court did not abuse its discretion in determining that the proposed evidence about compulsive gambling was irrelevant.

FOUCHA V. LOUISIANA, 504 U.S. 71 (1992)

Link to case: http://scholar.google.com/scholar_case?case=15775785182348520983

Question: Must an insanity acquittee be both mentally ill and dangerous for a state to justify continued hospitalization?

Answer: Yes.

Mr. Foucha was committed to a Louisiana psychiatric hospital as an insanity acquittee. Under Louisiana law, after the hospital committee recommends that the acquittee be released, the trial court must hold a hearing to determine whether the acquittee is a danger to himself or others. The statute allowed the acquittee to be returned to the hospital for further treatment simply on the basis of dangerousness. Mr. Foucha was retained in the hospital after a psychiatrist testified at his hearing that although Mr. Foucha was not mentally ill, he continued to exhibit symptoms of antisocial personality disorder that rendered him dangerous. On appeal, the Louisiana Supreme Court confirmed the judgment; Mr. Foucha appealed. The U.S. Supreme Court reversed, reasoning that because Mr. Foucha was no longer mentally ill, it would be a violation of his due process right (as interpreted by earlier case law) to continue to hold him as a mentally ill person. The Court also found that the statute violated the Equal Protection Clause, since it discriminates against insanity acquittees who would be retained although they do not differ from other criminals who may be dangerous but whose confinement would be subject to the rules of temporary pretrial detention and the expectation of definite release at the end of their sentence.

CLARK V. ARIZONA, 548 U.S. 735 (2006)

Link to case: http://caselaw.lp.findlaw.com/scripts/getcase.pl?navby=case&court=us&vol=548&page=735

Question: Can a state restrict evidence of mental illness at the time of a crime from being used as a mens rea defense (as opposed to legal insanity)?

Answer: Yes.

Question: Are states with insanity defense statutes constitutionally required to include a volitional prong?

Answer: No.

Eric Michael Clark shot and killed a police officer in Flagstaff, Arizona, and then argued at trial that he had a history of schizophrenia that included delusions that the police officer was an alien who was trying to kill him. He argued that he was therefore not guilty of the statutorily defined crime of intent to kill a police officer, and that he was also legally insane. The judge, in accordance with the Arizona penal code, denied Mr. Clark's attempt to plead lack of intent and restricted his mental illness defense to legal insanity. Mr. Clark sought to vacate the judgment based on the argument that the Arizona statute was unconstitutional because it only included the cognitive knowledge (right vs. wrong) prong. Mr. Clark also argued that the judge violated his due process rights when he applied an Arizona case (also known as the "Mott rule") that did not allow evidence of mental illness for the purposes of insanity to be used to rebut evidence of criminal intent. The trial court denied Mr. Clark's request to vacate, and the Arizona Court of Appeals agreed. The U.S. Supreme Court noted that states have varying standards for legal insanity and that there is no constitutional right to the volitional (could not control oneself) prong. With reference to the "Mott rule," the Court reasoned that Arizona made a reasonable decision to confine the consideration of evidence of mental disease and incapacity to the insanity defense so that it can preserve a legal presumption of sanity and the requirement that a defendant prove his insanity.

CHAPTER 26

Prisoners' Rights

OMAR KHAN, REBECCA LEWIS, AND BIPIN SUBEDI

ESTELLE V. GAMBLE, 429 U.S. 97 (1976)

Link to case: http://scholar.google.com/scholar_case?case=4755107314332030951

Question: Is medical negligence enough to prove a constitutional violation of a prisoner's right to treatment?

Answer: No.

J. W. Gamble was a Texas Department of Corrections (DOC) inmate who was injured when a bale of cotton fell on him while he was unloading a truck. He was diagnosed with "lower back strain." Mr. Gamble was evaluated 17 times for back pain and cardiac problems over the next 3 months. He was excused from work duties, but prison staff did not follow through with other medical orders. He received medication with little benefit. After several months Mr. Gamble was medically cleared, but he refused to go to work due to ongoing pain. He was placed in administrative segregation, then solitary confinement. Mr. Gamble sued W. J. Estelle, director of the DOC, and other staff members, stating that their "refusal" to provide care violated his Eighth Amendment right against cruel and unusual punishment. The district court dismissed the complaint, the U.S. Court of Appeals for the Fifth Circuit reversed/remanded, and the U.S. Supreme Court agreed to hear the case. The Court ruled that prison officials must demonstrate "deliberate indifference"—defined as intentionally denying/delaying access to medical care—for refusal of services to be considered cruel and unusual. Mr. Gamble's care may have been negligent, but it was not necessarily deliberately indifferent. The case was remanded with instructions to apply the above standard to the others named in the suit.

VITEK V. JONES, 445 U.S. 480 (1980)

Link to case: http://scholar.google.com/scholar_case?case=12392576224835810750

Question: Is a prisoner constitutionally entitled to procedural protections before involuntary transfer to a psychiatric hospital for treatment?

Answer: Yes.

In May 1974, Larry Jones was convicted of robbery and sentenced to 3 to 9 years in the Nebraska state penitentiary. He was transferred to the penitentiary hospital in January 1975, 2 days after which he set fire to his mattress, severely burned himself, and required treatment for the burns at a private hospital. After receiving treatment for the burns, Mr. Jones was transferred to Lincoln Regional Center (a state psychiatric hospital) in accordance with Nebraska law requiring a designated physician or psychologist to find that Mr. Jones suffered from a "mental disease or defect" and could not "be given proper treatment" within the correctional institution. Mr. Jones challenged the constitutionality of this statute; the district court agreed and declared the transfer unconstitutional. The U.S. District Court opined that the transfer infringed on Mr. Jones's liberty interest protected by the Due Process Clause of the Fourteenth Amendment and had "stigmatizing" consequences beyond those imposed by incarceration for conviction of a crime. In March 1980, the U.S. Supreme Court affirmed the district court decision requiring the state to abide by the following procedures before transfer of a prisoner to a mental hospital: written notice to the prisoner, a hearing allowing for presentation of evidence and testimony, an independent decision maker, a written statement by the fact-finder, and legal counsel for the prisoner.

WASHINGTON V. HARPER, 494 U.S. 210 (1990)

Link to case: http://scholar.google.com/scholar_case?case=13274222040240404814

Question: Is a judicial hearing about medication required to satisfy due process for a dangerous, convicted prisoner refusing psychiatric medication?

Answer: No.

Walter Harper was incarcerated in the Washington state penal system. On two occasions, he was transferred to the Special Offender Center (SOC), a state institute for convicted felons with serious mental illness. While there, he was required to take antipsychotic medications against his will pursuant to an SOC policy, which provided that a hospital committee review the need for involuntary medication. Mr. Harper filed suit, claiming that the lack of a judicial hearing about involuntary medication violated his due process rights under the Fourteenth Amendment. The trial court rejected his claim. The Washington State Supreme Court reversed and remanded, concluding that a judicial hearing was necessary. The U.S. Supreme Court granted certiorari and noted the following: (1) there is a legitimate state interest in combating danger posed by a violent mentally ill inmate, and (2) there is little dispute that proper use of medications is an effective means of treating mental illness. The Court held that the SOC policy satisfied both substantive and procedural due process and reversed the Washington State Supreme Court ruling. The Court wrote that liberty interests might be better served by allowing the decision to medicate to be made by medical professionals rather than a judge. The SOC policy fulfilled procedural due process by mandating notice of a hearing, the right to representation by a disinterested adviser, and the right to appeal to the state court.

RIGGINS V. NEVADA, 504 U.S. 127 (1992)

Link to case: http://scholar.google.com/scholar_case?case=7905994277524677132

Question: Can a person standing trial be forced to take antipsychotic medication without a determination that it is both medically appropriate and the least intrusive option?

Answer: No.

David Riggins was charged with murder. He was prescribed thioridazine for auditory hallucinations and was found competent to stand trial. The defense moved to suspend thioridazine during the trial, arguing that the medication's effects on Mr. Riggins's demeanor would affect the jury's opinion of him and therefore deny him a fair trial. The district court denied the motion. Mr. Riggins presented the insanity defense and was convicted and sentenced to death. He appealed, arguing that the forced administration of thioridazine violated his right to assist in his defense, and that the state should have demonstrated medical need for the treatment as well as that there were no less intrusive means. The Nevada Supreme Court affirmed his conviction and death sentence. The U.S. Supreme Court granted certiorari and reversed the decision. Referring to *Washington v. Harper*, the Court found that forcing antipsychotic medications on a convicted prisoner is impermissible without overriding justification and a determination of medical appropriateness. The Court found that the Fourteenth Amendment affords at least as much protection to persons standing trial as to those convicted and sentenced. It noted that Nevada would have satisfied due process if the state had demonstrated that thioridazine was medically appropriate, the least intrusive option, and essential for the safety of Mr. Riggins or others. The Court did not directly address whether a person may be medicated forcibly for the purpose of maintaining competence to stand trial.

FARMER V. BRENNAN, 511 U.S. 825 (1994)

Link to case: http://scholar.google.com/scholar_case?case=2417836767044325448

Question: Does the "deliberate indifference" standard outlined in *Estelle v. Gamble* require actual knowledge of risk by prison officials?

Answer: Yes.

Dee Farmer, a male-to-female preoperative transsexual, was convicted of credit card fraud and sentenced to federal prison in 1986. In 1989, Ms. Farmer was transferred to a higher-security facility for disciplinary reasons. Following this transfer, Ms. Farmer was allegedly beaten and raped by a male inmate in her cell. Ms. Farmer filed a civil suit alleging an Eighth Amendment violation against prison officials for being deliberately indifferent with regard to protecting her safety. The U.S. District Court granted summary judgment to the prison officials that was affirmed by the U.S. Court of Appeals for the Seventh Circuit. The U.S. Supreme Court heard the case and decided that prison officials may be held liable for deliberate indifference only if they are aware of a "substantial risk of serious harm" and they "disregard that risk by failing to take reasonable measures to abate it." According to the ruling, deliberate indifference is somewhere above negligence but below purposeful or knowledgeable harm, and the appropriate test for this case was determined to be that of "subjective recklessness."

The U.S. Supreme Court vacated the decision and remanded the case for further review.

SELL V. U.S., 539 U.S. 166 (2003)

Link to case: http://scholar.google.com/scholar_case?case=10071406451224631321

Question: Can antipsychotic drugs be forced on a criminal defendant in order to restore competence to stand trial?

Answer: Yes.

Charles Sell was a dentist with a psychotic disorder who was indicted for health care fraud and attempted murder in Missouri. Dr. Sell was found incompetent to stand trial and, while hospitalized, refused antipsychotic medication. The magistrate authorized forced administration of antipsychotic medication, finding that Dr. Sell was dangerous. The district court found the magistrate's dangerousness finding erroneous but concluded that medication was necessary to render Dr. Sell competent to stand trial and, therefore, necessary to serve the government interest in adjudicating his case. The U.S. Court of Appeals for the Eighth Circuit affirmed, finding that the government had an essential interest in bringing Dr. Sell to trial and that the treatment was medically appropriate. The U.S. Supreme Court granted certiorari and found that the Constitution permits the government to involuntarily administer antipsychotic medications to mentally ill defendants in order to restore competence to stand trial if (1) "important government interests are at stake" (i.e., the crime is a serious one against person or property), (2) the treatment is medically appropriate, (3) the treatment is in fact likely to "render the defendant competent," (4) the treatment is "substantially unlikely to have side effects that will interfere significantly with the defendant's ability to assist counsel," and (5) taking account of less intrusive alternatives, the treatment is necessary to further governmental trial-related interests. Because the original decisions reviewed by the lower federal courts were based only on Sell's dangerousness, the Court concluded that there was insufficient evidence to apply the necessary constitutional criteria it established. Consequently, the case was remanded for further consideration.

BROWN V. PLATA, 131 S. CT. 1910 (2011)

Link to case: http://scholar.google.com/scholar_case?case=4913884626785841743

Question: Was a special district court ruling to drastically reduce the inmate population in California's prison system necessary and authorized by Congress?

Answer: Yes.

Brown v. Plata is a consolidation of two class action cases brought against the governor of California (Brown) alleging violations of Eighth Amendment rights in the California prison system. *Coleman v. Brown*, filed in 1990, involves a class of prisoners with serious mental disorders, and *Plata v. Brown*, filed in 2001, involves a class of prisoners with serious medical conditions. In 2008, after years of failures of remedial plans related to both cases and conditions that did not meet the minimally adequate standard and in accordance with the Prison Litigation Reform Act (PLRA) of 1995, a three-judge district court was convened to assess whether overcrowding was the source of the constitutional violations. If so, according to the PLRA, the court needed to find by clear and convincing evidence that there was no appropriate remedy other than reducing the prison population and that such a remedy must be narrowly tailored and issued only after strong consideration of the impact on public safety. The court determined that for more than a decade the California prison system had been operating at almost double the capacity that it was designed to accommodate. As a result, the system was unable to meet the basic health needs of its inmates. The court ordered that the prison population be reduced to 137.5% of its designed capacity within 2 years. The State of California appealed the decision, but the U.S. Supreme Court affirmed, finding that the district court was convened appropriately and that overcrowding was the primary cause of the substandard prison health care conditions.

CHAPTER 27

Death Penalty

TARA STRAKA

ESTELLE V. SMITH, 451 U.S. 454 (1981)

Link to case: http://scholar.google.com/scholar_case?case=3874052948546256691

Question: Is information gathered as part of a pretrial psychiatric evaluation admissible during the sentencing phase of a death penalty case?

Answer: No.

Ernest Smith sought habeas corpus relief after receiving a death sentence for murder. Mr. Smith challenged the way psychiatric evidence about him had been obtained and used against him at sentencing. When Mr. Smith was indicted for murder and Texas announced its intention to seek the death penalty, the trial court ordered a psychiatric examination for competency to stand trial. Dr. James Grigson evaluated Mr. Smith without defense counsel's awareness and found him fit to proceed. Mr. Smith was tried by a jury and convicted. During the penalty phase, Dr. Grigson was called as a prosecution witness and testified about Mr. Smith's potential for future dangerousness based on his pretrial examination. The U.S. Court of Appeals, Fifth Circuit found that Mr. Smith's protection from self-incrimination (Fifth Amendment) and his right to counsel (Sixth amendment) had been violated. The U.S. Supreme Court agreed. The Court noted that the prosecution used Mr. Smith's "own statement, unwittingly made without an awareness that he was assisting the State's efforts to obtain the death penalty."

AKE V. OKLAHOMA, 470 U.S. 68 (1985)

Link to case: http://scholar.google.com/scholar_case?case=1904002630366313299

Question: Does the state have to provide access to a psychiatric evaluation for an indigent defendant in a case where legal insanity is at issue?

Answer: Yes.

Glen Ake was arrested for murder. At arraignment, his behavior was so bizarre that the judge ordered a competency evaluation. He was found incompetent to stand trial and was committed to the state psychiatric hospital for restoration. Mr. Ake subsequently pled insanity and requested that a psychiatrist be appointed at state expense to evaluate his state of mind at the time of the offense. The judge denied the request, and the defense called the treating psychiatrists from the state hospital. However, none of them could testify to Mr. Ake's mental state at the time of the offense because they had not evaluated such during his treatment. He was found guilty and sentenced to death, which was upheld on appeal. The U.S. Supreme Court found that it is a violation of the Fourteenth Amendment's guarantee of due process for the state to deny the defendant a psychiatric consultant "who will conduct an appropriate examination and assist in evaluation, preparation, and presentation of the defense." The Court remanded the case for a new trial. However, the Court also ruled that the defense was not necessarily entitled to a consultant of his choosing.

FORD V. WAINWRIGHT, 477 U.S. 399 (1986)

Link to case: http://scholar.google.com/scholar_case?case=7904262174469084060

Question: Can an insane prisoner be executed?

Answer: No.

In 1974, Alvin Ford was convicted of murdering a police officer and sentenced to death. He became delusional after sentencing. Two psychiatrists hired by the defense found him incompetent to be executed, but three psychiatrists appointed by the governor found him competent based on a 30-minute interview. No adversarial hearing or cross-examination of any psychiatrist was permitted, and the governor did not acknowledge reports submitted by the defense counsel. Without explanation, the governor signed the death warrant. Mr. Ford filed a habeas corpus petition alleging that the procedures under which his competency to be executed was upheld were unconstitutional. After the 11th Circuit Court of Appeals affirmed the sentence, Mr. Ford appealed to the U.S. Supreme Court. The Court found the Florida statute governing this competency determination was unconstitutional because it allowed the finding to be carried out by the executive branch. The Court opined that a "full and fair hearing" was required, noting that this level of due process was required because execution of the insane is inherently offensive and does not meet the goals of either retribution or deterrence.

PAYNE V. TENNESSEE, 501 U.S. 808 (1991)

Link to case: http://scholar.google.com/scholar_case?case=7795411704028596196

Question: Is the inclusion of victim impact statements during the sentencing phase of a capital trial a violation of the Eighth Amendment?

Answer: No.

Pervis Tyrone Payne was convicted of capital murder after a brutal attack on a family in which he murdered a mother and her 2-year-old daughter and severely wounded her 3-year-old son. At sentencing, the 3-year-old victim's grandmother testified for the state about how the boy was affected by the crime and the loss of his mother and sister. Mr. Payne appealed his death sentence, claiming that his Eighth Amendment rights had been violated by the state's presentation of the grandmother's testimony. The state supreme court ruled that victim impact evidence can be presented; the U.S. Supreme Court affirmed. The U.S. Supreme Court had previously ruled in *Booth v. Maryland* and *South Carolina v. Gathers* that such evidence could not be presented at a capital trial sentencing phase. However, the Court now noted that stare decisis is not an "inexorable command," and "when governing decisions are unworkable or are badly reasoned, 'this Court has never felt constrained to follow precedent.'" It reasoned that the prior decision "unfairly weighted the scales in a capital trial" by preventing the state from countering mitigating evidence presented by the defense. It noted that victim impact statements show the specific harm caused by the crime, which aids the jury in assessing the defendant's moral culpability and also shows the victim as a unique individual.

STATE V. PERRY, 610 SO. 2D 746 (LA. 1992)

Link to case: http://scholar.google.com/scholar_case?case=12731842654315565192

Question: Can a state involuntarily treat a death row prisoner with antipsychotic drugs to make him competent to be executed?

Answer: No.

Michael Owen Perry, a man with a long history of mental illness and a diagnosis of schizophrenia, was convicted and sentenced to death for murdering his parents, two cousins, and a nephew. His conviction was affirmed on appeal; however, the court ordered an evaluation of his competence to be executed. The trial court found him competent and ordered that he continue treatment with haloperidol to maintain his competence—even if that meant treating him over his objection. Mr. Perry appealed, but the U.S. Supreme Court sent the case back to the state for consideration pursuant to the standards it set under *Washington v. Harper*, that is, the balancing of an inmate's liberty interests in avoiding unwanted treatment, his medical need for that treatment, and the state's interest in prison safety. After the trial court reinstated treatment over objection, the Louisiana Supreme Court stayed the order. It held that forcing drugs merely to facilitate execution "does not constitute medical treatment but is antithetical to the basic principles of the healing arts" and that doing so would violate the inmate's right to privacy and amount to cruel and unusual punishment under the Louisiana state constitution. Therefore, the state may not medicate incompetent death row prisoners over their objections simply for the purpose of restoring the prisoner to competence for execution.

ATKINS V. VIRGINIA, 536 U.S. 304 (2002)

Link to case: http://caselaw.lp.findlaw.com/scripts/getcase.pl?navby=case&court=us&vol=536&page=304

Question: Does the Constitution prohibit the execution of a person with mental retardation?

Answer: Yes.

Daryl Atkins was convicted of murder and sentenced to death for abducting, robbing, and shooting a man. At the sentencing phase, the defense introduced a psychologist who testified that Atkins was mildly mentally retarded and had an IQ of 59. The Virginia Supreme Court affirmed the death sentence based on *Penry v. Lynaugh*, a 1989 U.S. Supreme Court case that allowed for the execution of individuals with mental retardation. In the *Atkins* case, the U.S. Supreme Court overruled this prior 1989 holding, now finding that executing mentally retarded prisoners was inconsistent with the "evolving standards of decency" that define what is considered "cruel and unusual punishment" under the Eighth Amendment. The Court noted that after the *Penry* case, a large number of states since 1989 had passed laws prohibiting the execution of the mentally retarded, and polls indicated that the majority of Americans were opposed to their execution. In addition, the Court reasoned that "executing the mentally retarded serves neither to deter others nor to mete out retribution appropriate for the lower level of culpability."

ROPER V. SIMMONS, 543 U.S. 551 (2005)

Link to case: http://caselaw.lp.findlaw.com/scripts/getcase.pl?navby=case&court=us&vol=543&page=551

Question: Does the Constitution prohibit the execution of an individual who committed a capital crime when he was under the age of 18?

Answer: Yes.

Christopher Simmons was 17 years old when he and an accomplice abducted a woman and threw her off a bridge to her death. Mr. Simmons had planned the crime in advance, stating that he wanted to "murder someone," and then bragged about it afterward. Mr. Simmons was tried as an adult and sentenced to death. The Missouri Supreme Court affirmed the conviction and sentence. However, Mr. Simmons used the "evolving standards of decency" reasoning of the intervening U.S. Supreme Court decision in *Atkins v. Virginia* and filed a second appeal against Donald Roper, the superintendent of Potosi Correctional Center, with the Missouri Supreme Court. The Missouri court agreed with Mr. Simmons despite U.S. Supreme Court precedent in *Stanford v. Kentucky* that the minimum age for capital punishment was 16. In a 5–4 decision, The U.S. Supreme Court agreed with the Missouri court (and Mr. Simmons), holding that the execution of an individual for a crime committed before the age of 18 was a violation of the Eighth and Fourteenth Amendments. Similar to *Atkins*, the Court based its opinion on the fact that the majority of states (and international law) did not permit the execution of juveniles. The Court noted that the scientific community viewed adolescence as a period of poor decision-making, developmental immaturity, and susceptibility to peer pressure, all of which rendered adolescents less culpable than adults and therefore not deserving of the ultimate penalty (i.e., death).

PANETTI V. QUARTERMAN, 127 S. CT. 2842 (2007)

Link to case: http://scholar.google.com/scholar_case?case=2278250008123789539

Question: Are a "rational understanding" and a "factual awareness" necessary for a person to be found competent to be executed?

Answer: Yes.

Scott Panetti was sentenced to death for the murder of his estranged wife's parents. Mr. Panetti asked for a stay of execution, claiming that he was not competent to be executed. Nathaniel Quarterman was the director of the Correctional Institutions Division of the Texas Department of Criminal Justice. Mr. Panetti was examined, and the state court found him competent, without a hearing. On appeal, the U.S. Court of Appeals for the Fifth Circuit affirmed the finding, reasoning that although Mr. Panetti believed the real reason for his execution was to prevent him from preaching the gospel, he knew the state was executing him for murder. According to the court, this met the *Ford* standard for competency to be executed. The U.S. Supreme Court then reversed the Fifth Circuit holding. It stated that the *Ford* case required consideration of both Mr. Panetti's factual awareness that he was being executed and his "rational understanding" of the reasons for the execution. The Court also found that the procedures for evaluating Mr. Panetti's claim of incapacity were inadequate. However, the Court did not outline a specific standard for competency to be executed.

CHAPTER 28

Sex Offenders

LI-WEN G. LEE

SPECHT V. PATTERSON, 386 U.S. 605 (1967)

Link to case: http://scholar.google.com/scholar_case?case=3723552257968594646

Question: Can a person convicted under one statute be sentenced under a different statute without a new hearing?

Answer: No.

Francis Specht was convicted in Colorado for indecent liberties, a sex offense with a maximum 10-year sentence. Without notice and full hearing, he was sentenced under the Sex Offenders Act to an indeterminate term of 1 day to life. The act could be applied to convicted sex offenders found to be either a threat to the public if at large or a habitual offender and mentally ill. The procedure under the act required a psychiatric examination and report to be submitted to a court but did not include a full hearing. There was no opportunity to confront witnesses or to access hearsay evidence. Mr. Specht filed a habeas corpus petition for his release. Both the Colorado Supreme Court and then the U.S. Court of Appeals for the 10th Circuit rejected his petition. Mr. Specht then appealed to the U.S. Supreme Court. The Court held that commitment proceedings, whether civil or criminal, are still subject to the constitutional guarantees of the Fourteenth Amendment. The Court noted that the determination and sentencing under the act is a criminal punishment, despite its intention to prevent future harm rather than for retribution. As a result, due process protections are required, including the presence of counsel and the opportunity to be heard, to be confronted with adverse witnesses, to cross-examine, and to offer evidence.

ALLEN V. ILLINOIS, 478 U.S. 364 (1986)

Link to case: http://scholar.google.com/scholar_case?case=946918575027007848

Question: Does the Fifth Amendment protection against self-incrimination apply to Illinois's Sexual Dangerous Persons Act?

Answer: No.

Terry Allen was charged in Illinois with unlawful restraint and deviate sexual assault. The state sought to have him found a sexually dangerous person under the Illinois Sexually Dangerous Persons Act, a finding that requires proving the existence of a mental disorder for more than 1 year and a propensity to commit sexual assaults. In accordance with the act, two psychiatrists whose testimony was presented at trial examined Mr. Allen. He was found to be a sexually dangerous person and then appealed on the basis that the psychiatric testimony included information elicited from him in violation of his privilege against self-incrimination. The Appellate Court of Illinois for the Third District agreed with Mr. Allen, but the Supreme Court of Illinois upheld the determination. The U.S. Supreme Court then heard the case and agreed with the state. It found that although the act could only be applied if criminal charges were already filed, the act itself was not criminal but civil in nature because the goal was to provide treatment rather than punishment. It found that the provision of care in a maximum security facility also providing care to convicts did not establish punishment over treatment. In addition, the provision of some due process safeguards by the act did not turn the act into a criminal proceeding requiring the full range of due process protections. The Court further noted that the Fourteenth Amendment guarantee of due process does not require application of the Fifth Amendment privilege against self-incrimination.

IN RE YOUNG AND CUNNINGHAM, 857 P.2D 989 (1993)

Link to case: http://www.mrsc.org/wa/courts/index_dtSearch.html

Question: Is the Washington State sexually violent predator statute a criminal law?

Answer: No.

Andre Brigham Young was incarcerated after conviction for rape and had a history of committing other rapes. One day prior to his release, the state filed for commitment under the Washington sexually violent predator statute, the Community Protection Act of 1990. Vance Russell Cunningham was convicted of an unrelated rape; he also had a history of committing prior sexual offenses. In Mr. Cunningham's case, the state filed for commitment several months after he had been released from prison. Mr. Young and Mr. Cunningham appealed to the Supreme Court of Washington and argued that the statute violated the double jeopardy clause and the prohibition against ex post facto laws. The court concluded that the statute was civil and that therefore the criminal protections of double jeopardy and ex post facto laws did not apply. It noted that commitment requires a mental disorder leading to the commission of violent sexual offenses and that committed persons are treated in a psychiatric facility and released as soon as they are no longer dangerous. Mr. Young and Mr. Cunningham also argued that substantive and procedural due process were violated in a number of ways. On these issues, the court found that a defendant must be permitted to appear in court within 72 hours to contest probable cause, the state was required to show acute dangerousness for defendants not incarcerated, least restrictive alternatives must be considered, and jury unanimity was required at the beyond a reasonable doubt threshold.

KANSAS V. HENDRICKS, 521 U.S. 346 (1997)

Link to case: http://scholar.google.com/scholar_case?case=3660172212792959574

Question: Does the procedure for civil commitment established by the Kansas Sexually Violent Predator (SVP) Act violate principles of due process, double jeopardy, and ex post facto?

Answer: No.

Leroy Hendricks was convicted of taking indecent liberties with two 13-year-old boys and was then incarcerated. Shortly before his release, the state sought to civilly confine Mr. Hendricks as a sexually violent predator under the Kansas SVP Act. During his trial to determine whether he qualified as a sexually violent predator, Mr. Hendricks testified about his lengthy history of sexual offenses against children. He further admitted to abusing children whenever not confined, and while he expressed the hope to not offend against children again, he stated that the only guarantee was "to die." He agreed with the diagnosis of pedophilia, acknowledged that he was not cured, and further opined that the treatment was ineffective. He was found to be a sexually violent predator and to have a "mental abnormality" qualifying him for confinement under the act. Mr. Hendricks claimed that the act violated the due process, double jeopardy, and ex post facto clauses of the Constitution. The Kansas Supreme Court agreed that "mental abnormality" did not meet the standard of a mental illness for involuntary commitment purposes; the State of Kansas appealed to the U.S. Supreme Court. The Court reversed the appellate decision by ruling that the definition of "mental abnormality" in the act satisfied "substantive" due process requirements in that the act requires a precommitment finding of dangerousness linked to a "mental abnormality." The specific term "mental illness" is not required. The Court further found that lack of effective treatment did not make the act unconstitutional and that double jeopardy and ex post facto prohibitions do not apply because the act is civil in nature.

MCKUNE V. LILE, 536 U.S. 24 (2002)

Link to case: http://scholar.google.com/scholar_case?case=16143402596203476658

Question: Does incentivizing participation during incarceration in the Kansas Sexual Abuse Treatment Program (SATP), which requires admitting past offenses, violate the Fifth Amendment privilege against self-incrimination?

Answer: No.

Robert Lile was convicted of rape, aggravated sodomy, and aggravated kidnaping despite his claim that the sexual activity was consensual. Before release from prison, he was ordered to participate in the SATP, which requires discussion and acceptance of responsibility of the crime(s) of conviction as well as details of prior sexual activities, including uncharged criminal offenses. This information is not privileged, although at the time Mr. Lile's case was heard, there was no incriminating evidence released under the SATP. Refusal to participate in the program would result in loss of certain privileges and transfer to a maximum security prison. Mr. Lile refused to participate on the grounds that the consequences of nondisclosure were so significant that they constituted compelled self-incrimination that would violate his Fifth Amendment privilege. He sought an injunction to prevent loss of privileges and transfer to a more secure facility. The district court agreed about the Fifth Amendment violation claim, and the U.S. Court of Appeals for the Tenth Circuit affirmed. The U.S. Supreme Court did not agree, however, and found that the program did not violate Mr. Lile's Fifth Amendment right as along as (1) the program served a legitimate penological objective, (2) the consequences also had a rehabilitative function (i.e., teach that actions have consequences), and (3) the consequences were not so severe as to be coercive.

KANSAS V. CRANE, 534 U.S. 407 (2002)

Link to case:
http://scholar.google.com/scholar_case?case=11856713111605024563

Question: Does the ruling in *Kansas v. Hendricks* require the state to prove that a dangerous individual is completely unable to control his behavior?

Answer: No.

Michael Crane was convicted of a sexual offense, and the state pursued civil commitment hearings under the Kansas SVP Act. A psychiatric witness for the state diagnosed him with exhibitionism and antisocial personality disorder, and the trial court ordered his commitment without a finding regarding whether he could control his dangerous behavior. Mr. Crane's commitment was overturned on appeal to the Kansas Supreme Court based on a ruling that Mr. Crane did not meet the *Hendricks* requirement of proof that a dangerous individual is completely unable to control his behavior. Kansas appealed to the U.S. Supreme Court with the argument that the interpretation of the appellate court was too rigid. The U.S. Supreme Court determined that a complete lack of control was not necessary to be committed as a sexually violent predator. It commented on the importance of including some volitional criteria in order to distinguish dangerous offenders subject to civil commitment from those appropriately addressed exclusively through criminal proceedings. Because lack of control is not demonstrable with "mathematical precision," the Court noted that serious difficulty controlling behavior was adequate for SVP determinations.

U.S. V. COMSTOCK, 560 U.S. 126 (2010)

Link to case: http://scholar.google.com/scholar_case?case=11856713111605024563

Question: Can Congress enact legislation to civilly commit convicted, mentally ill, sexually violent federal prisoners beyond their schedule release date?

Answer: Yes.

In 2006, the U.S. government instituted postincarceration civil commitment proceedings against five men convicted of sexual offenses. Three of the men had been charged with possession of child pornography, and the other two with sexual abuse of a minor. The government sought to confine them pursuant to Federal Statute 4248, which allowed for the indefinite confinement of mentally ill, sexually dangerous federal prisoners beyond the date they would otherwise be released, with "mental illness" defined as having a disorder that would make it difficult to refrain from "sexually violent conduct or child molestation." The men opposed their commitment, making double jeopardy, ex post facto, equal protection, and due process claims (including that the standard of proof should be beyond a reasonable doubt). They also claimed that Congress had exceeded its powers in enacting the civil commitment statute. The district court dismissed the case, and the U.S. Court of Appeals for the Fourth Circuit affirmed the dismissal. The U.S. Supreme Court granted certiorari about the congressional power issue and found that Congress had the power to enact this civil commitment statute. It noted that while the scope of the federal government was restricted by the Constitution, Congress did have the power to enact legislation that was "necessary and proper" and "rationally related" to the implementation of a constitutionally enumerated power (see Article I of the Constitution), in this case continuing a long-standing policy of providing care and control of individuals who may be at risk to third parties.

CHAPTER 29

Questions on Criminal Law and Incarceration

QUESTIONS

1. In its decision in *North Carolina v. Alford*, the U.S. Supreme Court affirmed which of the following statements?
   A. The Fourteenth Amendment requires that defendants retain their right to a guilty plea despite the advice of competent counsel.
   B. Mens rea need not be considered in cases of clearly premeditated murder.
   C. If the principal motivation behind a guilty plea is fear of death, the plea in invalidated.
   D. The standard for a plea is whether that plea is a "voluntary and intelligent" choice among one's options.
   E. Because the local North Carolina court issued the incorrect jury instructions, Alford's guilty plea should not have been accepted.

2. The U.S. Supreme Court has ruled that executing juveniles or the mentally retarded is a violation of which constitutional amendment?
   A. First
   B. Fifth
   C. Sixth
   D. Eighth
   E. Fourteenth

3. Which of the following statements is most accurate regarding diminished capacity defenses?
   A. They are required by the Due Process Clause of the U.S. Constitution.
   B. They cannot be advanced by *pro se* defendants.
   C. They are unrelated to issues of intent and mens rea.
   D. Their use and relevance are the purview of each state.
   E. They are unavailable to defendants opting for trial by jury.

4. A frequently cited basis for U.S. Supreme Court decisions finding that involuntary, postincarceration sexually violent predator commitment programs do not constitute criminal sanctions is:
   A. Involuntary commitments do not extend past the period of parole supervision after incarceration mandated during the sentencing phase of the criminal proceedings.
   B. Involuntary commitment is for the purpose of treatment rather than punishment.
   C. Involuntary commitment is for those individuals convicted of sexual offenses who failed to complete sex offender treatment during incarceration.
   D. Convicted sex offenders have both committed criminal acts and suffer from a mental disorder and therefore require both punishment and treatment.
   E. Involuntary commitment requires a showing that sexual offense recidivism is more likely than not after release from incarceration.

5. Is a mentally ill prisoner entitled to a judicial hearing before he receives treatment over objection?
   A. Yes. Mentally ill convicted prisoners need to be protected from prison-associated health care professionals, and a judicial hearing is therefore necessary to adjudicate treatment over objection.
   B. No. Mentally ill convicted prisoners do not have the right to refuse medically appropriate treatment.
   C. No. Mentally ill convicted prisoners have the right to refuse treatment, but an administrative review by medical professionals of the treatment refusal and the need for treatment over objection is sufficient to satisfy due process.
   D. Yes. Prisoners with mental illness are entitled to the same due process rights as individuals who are involuntarily committed to civilian hospitals.

6. The U.S. Supreme Court has ruled that a state is able to makes laws that:
   A. Punish people addicted to drugs with incarceration
   B. Punish people addicted to drugs with incarceration followed by forced treatment
   C. Force people addicted to drugs to undergo treatment
   D. Increase incarceration times for people addicted to drugs if they break another law
   E. Treat people addicted to drugs exactly as people who are not

7. Which of the following best illustrates the U.S. Supreme Court's use of the concept of an "evolving standard of decency"?
   A. *Roper v. Simmons* ruling against precedent set in *Stanford v. Kentucky*
   B. *Payne v. Tennessee* ruling against precedent set in *Booth v. Maryland*
   C. *Ford v. Wainwright* decision in keeping with the history of common law
   D. None of the above

8. *U.S. v. Comstock*, a case involving the civil commitment of a sex offender, was decided on the basis of:
   A. Procedural due process
   B. Substantive due process
   C. Double jeopardy
   D. Equal protection
   E. Congressional authority

9. What is the legal burden of proof in competence to stand trial hearings in federal court?
   A. Clear and convincing evidence
   B. Beyond a reasonable doubt
   C. Without due cause
   D. Preponderance of the evidence

10. In cases of extreme emotional disturbance (EED), the burden of proving the EED:
    A. is typically only to a preponderance of the evidence because these cases are normally civil in nature
    B. is a presumption in a criminal case and so needs to be proved in the negative by the state to beyond a reasonable doubt
    C. is closely related to whether the defendant is proposing a not guilty by reason of insanity plea

D. can constitutionally rest upon the defendant
E. need only apply if the murder occurred in the setting of a different violent crime, such as robbery

11. The primary reason given by the Court in establishing the affirmative need for the police to inform suspects of their rights was:
    A. Many defendants have borderline intelligence.
    B. First-time defendants cannot be assumed to know their rights.
    C. The application of specific constitutional rights varies from case to case.
    D. The inherently coercive nature of being in police custody
    E. Defendants are presumed incompetent to stand trial until proved otherwise.

12. A psychiatrist is asked by the prosecution to evaluate a capital defendant for competency to stand trial and to form an opinion about the defendant's future risk for dangerousness in case of a capital sentencing hearing. There is no notice given to defense counsel, and the psychiatrist does not explain the limits of confidentiality. According to the ruling in *Estelle v. Smith*, which best describes the way in which this defendant's constitutional rights have been violated?
    A. Fifth Amendment, because he did not know he could refuse, *and* Eighth Amendment, because prosecution is seeking the death penalty in a defendant who may not be competent for trial
    B. Sixth Amendment, because he did not know he could refuse examination
    C. Fifth Amendment, because he did not have access to counsel, *and* Sixth Amendment, because he did not know he could refuse
    D. Fifth Amendment, because he did not know he could refuse, *and* Sixth Amendment, because he did not have access to counsel
    E. Fifth Amendment, because he did not have access to counsel

13. Prior to the Insanity Defense Reform Act of 1984, if there was some evidence of mental illness, the burden of proof in federal court was on:
    A. The government to prove sanity by clear and convincing evidence
    B. The government to prove sanity by preponderance of the evidence
    C. The defendant to prove insanity beyond a reasonable doubt
    D. The defendant to prove insanity by clear and convincing evidence.

14. Consideration of competency at any time during a trial when sufficient doubt arises as to a defendant's current competence protects the defendant's right to:
    A. A fair trial
    B. Autonomy
    C. Freedom of speech
    D. Immunity

15. During participation in a sexual offender treatment program, the Fifth Amendment privilege against self-incrimination is:
    A. Protected by allowing persons to participate even if they have not acknowledged their offense(s) or provided a sexual history
    B. Protected by guaranteeing that disclosed information cannot be shared outside of treatment
    C. Not guaranteed because there is a legitimate goal of rehabilitation
    D. Not relevant because treatment occurs outside of the criminal justice system

16. Which of the following statements is most accurate regarding the Supreme Court's holding in *Montana v Egelhoff*?
    A. Voluntary intoxication was deemed a necessary consideration in criminal cases.
    B. The holding is not important to most jurisdictions, so it has had minimal impact on subsequent case law and practice.
    C. All states must offer charged defendants the option of pleading not guilty by reason of insanity.
    D. It affirmed that at least some jurisdictions can constitutionally preclude consideration of voluntary intoxication when trying a criminal defendant.
    E. All evidence, regardless of probative value, is required to be entertained by the trier of fact.

17. Which of the following statements is true?
    A. American Academy of Psychiatry and the Law (AAPL) ethical guidelines prohibit a psychiatrist from providing psychiatric treatment to a patient found incompetent to be executed.
    B. AAPL ethical guidelines prohibit psychiatrists from conducting examinations of competency to be sentenced in capital cases.
    C. American Medical Association (AMA) guidelines state that physicians should not participate in executions.
    D. American Psychiatric Association (APA) guidelines prohibit a psychiatrist from providing psychiatric treatment to a patient found incompetent to be executed.

E. The AMA states that testifying to medical aspects of aggravating or mitigating circumstances during the sentencing phase of a capital case constitutes physician participation in an execution.

18. The standard for a confession to be admissible is:
    A. Voluntary and knowing
    B. Informed consent
    C. Clear and convincing
    D. Competent
    E. Intelligent

19. What U.S. Supreme Court case first defined the criteria for competency to stand trial?
    A. *Drope v. Missouri*
    B. *Jackson v. Indiana*
    C. *Dusky v. U.S.*
    D. *Wilson v. U.S.*

20. An indigent defendant seeks to put forth an insanity defense, but the state denies his request to provide a psychiatric expert to examine his mental state at the time of the crime. According to *Ake v. Oklahoma*, what constitutional right has been violated?
    A. Fifth Amendment
    B. Sixth Amendment
    C. Eighth Amendment
    D. Fourteenth Amendment Due Process Clause
    E. Fourteenth Amendment Equal Protection Clause

21. Which of the following statements is most accurate regarding the decision of the Washington DC Court of Appeals in *Ibn-Tamas v. U.S.*?
    A. The "battered wife syndrome" is clearly a legitimate clinical entity and so should be considered by courts in cases involving alleged abuse.
    B. The "battered wife syndrome" is clearly not a legitimate clinical entity and so should not be considered by courts in cases involving alleged abuse.
    C. Expert testimony regarding the "battered wife syndrome" may be admissible, depending on the credentials of the expert and whether the testimony's probative value exceeds its potential prejudicial impact.
    D. The defense erred in selecting a psychologist as the expert because "battered wife syndrome" is more accurately placed in the purview of psychiatrists.

E. Clearly established victims of "battered wife syndrome" should have immediate and full exculpation if their violence was against the historical abuser.

22. Mr. Jones killed a man in a supermarket. He reports he could not conform his conduct to the law due to mental illness. In an American Law Institute (ALI) jurisdiction, with which of the following mental illnesses does Mr. Jones have the best chance of a successful NGRI defense?
    A. Pedophilia
    B. Antisocial personality disorder
    C. Fetal alcohol syndrome
    D. Post-traumatic stress disorder (PTSD)

23. The three-judge panel convened for *Brown v. Plata* to remedy the violation of prisoners' rights related to proper medical and mental health care was authorized under which congressional act?
    A. Employee Retirement Income Security Act (ERISA)
    B. Health Insurance Portability and Accountability Act (HIPPA)
    C. Prison Litigation Reform Act (PLRA)
    D. Mental Health Parity Act
    E. The Act of 1812

24. A successful diminished capacity defense:
    A. Can transfer a case from criminal to civil domain
    B. Frequently leads to full acquittal of charge
    C. Can be affirmatively placed despite clear lack of competence
    D. Can reduce a specific intent crime to a general intent crime
    E. Can originate from the prosecution

25. Mental disorder considerations in SVP commitment proceedings:
    A. Must be linked to sexually offending behaviors
    B. Are defined by the term "mental illness"
    C. Do not include personality disorders
    D. Are required to satisfy "procedural" due process requirements

26. A prison official who knowingly places a prisoner in a situation where the official is aware of a substantial risk of serious harm may be held liable for acting with:
    A. Nonmaleficence
    B. Deliberate indifference
    C. Failure to provide a comfortable environment
    D. Negligence
    E. Indifference

27. Which of the following cases addressed the issue of a mentally ill person's competence to be executed?
    A. *Atkins v. Virginia*
    B. *Roper v. Simmons*
    C. *Estelle v. Smith*
    D. *State v. Perry*
    E. *Ford v. Wainwright*

28. Which of the following statements is true regarding the involuntary treatment of a death row inmate with antipsychotic medication to restore his competence to be executed?
    A. The APA prohibits treatment of capital defendants who are incompetent to stand trial.
    B. In *State v. Perry*, the U.S. Supreme Court found that involuntary treatment with medication to restore competency represented cruel and unusual punishment.
    C. Federal law dictates that when an offender is convicted of a capital crime, he no longer maintains privacy rights that would allow him to refuse medical treatment.
    D. *Washington v. Harper* specifically addressed antipsychotic treatment refusal in death row inmates and found that it is unconstitutional for the state to treat over objection for the purpose of restoring competency.
    E. In *State v. Perry*, the court reasoned that forcing drugs merely to facilitate execution does not constitute medical treatment and instead violates the inmate's right to privacy and constitutes cruel and unusual punishment.

29. As a result of *Colorado v. Connelly*, it has been the case that a confession taken from police interrogation should be suppressed if:
    A. Miranda rights were not presented prior to the confession
    B. There was coercive police activity used in obtaining the police confession.
    C. The confession was not the product of "a rational intellect and free will."
    D. There was illegal search and seizure prior to the police interrogation.
    E. It is not promptly notarized following the confession.

30. Mr. Smith is a man with borderline intelligence who becomes depressed and is prescribed an antidepressant that leads to mania. He travels far away from his home, walks into a kindergarten, grabs a child, and announces to everyone that the child is the next Messiah. Mr. Smith is apprehended and charged with kidnapping. This is his first hospitalization and his first offense. He is found NGRI. At this point he has been treated and is asymptomatic. He requests a release. In his state, the statute requires that he be confined for 5 years prior to his first hearing because he was adjudicated mentally ill when he was found NGRI. He can argue that this statute violates:
    A. His right to treatment
    B. His substantive due process right
    C. Double jeopardy
    D. Equal protection

31. In *Vitek v. Jones*, the transfer of Mr. Jones to a mental hospital was declared unconstitutional because:
    A. It infringed on his rights prohibiting cruel and unusual punishment.
    B. It infringed on his right to due process under the Fourteenth Amendment.
    C. He was forced to acknowledge his mental illness.
    D. The receiving facility was unable to care for his basic medical needs.

32. The constitutional challenge to the procedure of police confessions in *Colorado v. Connelly* rests on which U.S. constitutional amendment?
    A. First
    B. Second
    C. Fourth
    D. Eighth
    E. Fourteenth

33. Which of the following was a major consideration in the decision in *Atkins v. Virginia*?
    A. Mental retardation does not affect an individual's culpability.
    B. Execution of mentally retarded offenders would provide a reasonable deterrent effect for other potential offenders with mental retardation.

C. Mentally retarded offenders may be less able to assist in their defense.
D. Very few states prohibit the execution of mentally retarded offenders.

34. Proof of lack of ability to control behavior in SVP commitment is:
    A. Not required if mental disorder or equivalent is shown because of the implied influence of mental disorder on volitional behavior
    B. Not required if the criminal history indicates repeated serious recidivistic behavior
    C. Required because there is a clear demarcation between emotional and volitional behavior
    D. Adequately established if there is proof of serious difficulty controlling behavior

35. Which of the following may be a reason that amnesia may render defendants incompetent?
    A. Inability to represent themselves *pro se*
    B. Inability to discuss proceedings rationally with their attorney
    C. Inability to remember all details of the alleged crime
    D. Ability to testify on their own behalf

36. What additional factor was added to the definition of the "deliberate indifference" standard in *Farmer v. Brennan*?
    A. Negligence
    B. Actual awareness of the risk of serious harm
    C. Disregard of the risk of harm
    D. Physical injury

37. Which of the following statements is true concerning the use of victim impact statements as decided in *Payne v. Tennessee*?
    A. Victim impact statements aid the jury in assessing moral culpability.
    B. Psychiatrists are prohibited from testifying about the psychological impact of a crime on the victim's family.
    C. The jury should decide a capital sentence based only on the character of the defendant and the circumstances of the crime.
    D. Victim impact statements contribute to arbitrary or capricious sentencing.
    E. The state does not have a legitimate interest in rebutting the mitigating evidence offered by the defense.

38. Which of the following NGRI defenses is most likely to succeed in a M'Naghten jurisdiction?
    A. A patient with obsessive-compulsive disorder who assaults someone on the street when an outdoor merchant attempts to sell her a piece of luggage she thinks is full of germs
    B. A patient with PTSD who shoots his girlfriend believing he was in the battlefield facing an undercover enemy combatant
    C. A patient with pathological gambling who could not stop himself from spending his employer's money at the casino
    D. A patient with pedophilic disorder who repeatedly masturbates in a children's park

39. The "necessary and proper" clause under which the statute in U.S. v. Comstock was determined to be constitutional can be found in which amendment?
    A. First
    B. Fifth
    C. Eighth
    D. Fourteenth
    E. None of the above

40. Mr. Dean, who has a history of schizoaffective disorder, went into a restaurant and shot all of the meat-eating diners. He was acutely psychotic at the time of the crime. In an ALI jurisdiction, which would he have to argue in order to get an NGRI verdict?
    A. At the time of the crime he believed that eating meat was morally wrong.
    B. At the time of the crime he was hearing auditory hallucinations telling him that God believes eating meat was wrong, and God was telling him to kill meat eaters in order to save these people from contracting and spreading deadly meat-born illnesses.
    C. At the time of the crime he believed that people who eat meat should be shot just like the animals that are shot for food.
    D. At the time of the crime he believed that God gave him special powers to eliminate those in the universe who are perpetrating crimes against animals.

41. The U.S. Supreme Court ruled that it is unconstitutional for a state to regulate drug abuse through:
    A. Criminal sanctions against the unauthorized manufacture, prescription, sale, purchase, or possession of narcotics within its borders

B. Compulsory treatment for those addicted to narcotics, with periods of involuntary confinement as part of a treatment program
C. Penal sanctions for a failure to comply with established compulsory treatment procedures
D. Public health education and efforts to ameliorate the economic and social conditions under which drug abuse flourishes
E. Imprisonment of an addict who travels through a state's jurisdiction

42. Legal challenges raised regarding commitment in SVP programs include:
    A. Double jeopardy
    B. Ex post facto lawmaking
    C. Substantive and procedural due process
    D. Fifth Amendment privilege against self-incrimination
    E. All of the above

43. In *People v. Patterson*, the New York Court of Appeals proposed which of the following arguments in its support of its state's law governing extreme emotional disturbance (EED) defenses?
    A. The law still required the state to prove all elements of the crime, despite placing the burden of proving the EED on the defense.
    B. The law had passed by a resounding majority in the senate and so should be offered wide latitude in interpretation.
    C. Because it was a state and not a federal law, it was not governed by the U.S. Constitution.
    D. Voluntary intoxication has always been accepted in common law and so should be incorporated into EED considerations.
    E. As a fundamental right, access to an EED defense is firmly rooted in the U.S. Constitution.

44. The case of *Powell v. Texas* (1968) led to the U.S. Supreme Court review of a statute for the alleged infliction of a cruel and unusual punishment. In this case, the Court ruled that Mr. Powell was rightfully convicted for:
    A. Being an alcoholic
    B. Being drunk in public
    C. Committing a murder while drunk
    D. Performing an unlawful act while drunk that was the product of a mental disease of defect
    E. Being unable to tell right from wrong when drunk

45. Can a pretrial detainee be treated over his objection for the purpose of restoring competence to stand trial?
    A. Yes, as long as the court finds that the patient is also dangerous.
    B. Yes, but only if certain criteria about medical appropriateness and governmental interests are met.
    C. No. Forcible medication can only be given against someone's will for purposes of treatment, not for competence to stand trial.
    D. No. Medications can never be given to a pretrial detainee against his will because the side effects might result in unfair trial prejudice.

46. Which of the following was cited as a reason to hold defendants to a different standard of competence for *pro se* representation than for competency to stand trial in *Indiana v. Edwards*?
    A. Mentally ill defendants are always incompetent.
    B. The variable quality of court-appointed legal personnel.
    C. The need to affirm the dignity of the defendant.
    D. The inherent inequality of the U.S. legal system.

47. *Brown v. Plata* involves a class of prisoners in California who:
    A. Alleged sexual abuse
    B. Alleged wrongful conviction
    C. Had serious medical problems
    D. Had serious mental health problems
    E. Had serious medical and mental health problems

48. Sex offender treatment programs during incarceration:
    A. Should not predicate prison privileges on program participation
    B. May require participants to take responsibility for the sexual offense leading to conviction
    C. Do not consider past sexual behaviors not associated with formal criminal history to be relevant
    D. Must be made available to those individuals who may be subject to SVP commitments

ANSWERS

1. **D**
   The U.S. Supreme Court, in its landmark decision in *North Carolina v. Alford*, held that Mr. Alford's plea, despite his protestation of

innocence, was appropriate because he was well counseled and had ample evidence supporting his guilt. It constituted a "knowing and intelligent" choice between the alternatives. The Court therefore felt that his guilty plea (which has since come to be known as an "Alford plea") was appropriately accepted by the lower court. One's right to a guilty plea is independent from the advice of counsel. Mens rea is a critical consideration in cases of murder. The *Alford* case refuted the contention that fear of death should invalidate a guilty plea. There were no issues of faulty jury instructions in the case.

2. **D**

    The Eighth Amendment protects against "cruel and unusual punishment." The U.S. Supreme Court cited the Eighth Amendment in holding that executing mentally retarded defendants (*Atkins v. Virginia*) or defendants who were juveniles at the time of their crime (*Roper v. Simmons*) is unconstitutional. The First Amendment protects freedom of speech. The Fifth Amendment provides the right to protection against self-incrimination. The Sixth Amendment provides the right to counsel. The Due Process Clause of the Fourteenth Amendment is used by the federal judiciary to make the Bill of Rights applicable to the states, and the Equal Protection Clause requires each state to provide equal protection under the law to similar classes of people in its jurisdiction.

3. **D**

    Diminished capacity defenses can, among other things, reduce a specific intent conviction (murder) to a general intent conviction (manslaughter). Because it is an affirmative defense, it originates with the defendant, not the prosecutor. It is unrelated to jurisdiction of charge and requires a competent defendant. While it is possible that a diminished capacity defense can lead to full charge acquittal (e.g., if there were no lesser charges based on the diminished capacity), this is rarely the case.

4. **B**

    The decisions in *Allen v. Illinois*, 478 U.S. 364 (1986), *In re Young and Cunningham*, 857 P.2d 989 (1993), and *Kansas v. Hendricks*, 521 U.S. 346 (1997) cite, in part, the goal of treatment. The role of treatment, even if in conjunction with incapacitation or as an ancillary goal, establishes sexually violent predator statutes as nonpunitive in nature and therefore subject to standards for civil, rather than criminal, proceedings. Commitments may extend until there is a showing that the confined person is no longer dangerous, independent of the duration of criminal sanctions. Completion, or not, of sex offender treatment during incarceration may be a consideration in mental abnormality and dangerousness considerations, but neither the SVP statutes nor court decisions specifically cite failure to complete sex offender treatment as a necessary criterion in determining civil commitment status. SVP acts have been found to address treatment needs rather than to serve as supplemental punishment to criminal sanctions. SVP statutes require a mental abnormality to be found, in addition to the showing of dangerousness.

5. **C**

 In *Washington v. Harper*, Mr. Harper was a prisoner at a state institution for convicted felons with serious mental illness. He refused medications, and the state institution followed its policy of a hospital committee review of the need for medications over objection. Mr. Harper filed suit, claiming that a judicial hearing with findings of substituted judgment was necessary. The U.S. Supreme Court ruled that the hospital review and using professional judgment regarding medications satisfied due process.

6. **C**

 In *Robinson v. California*, the U.S. Supreme Court ruled that people addicted to drugs could not be criminally punished for the "status" of being addicted (therefore A, B, and D are false). They could, however, be mandated to treatment in the interests of public health and regulating drug trafficking (therefore E is false). This allowed laws specifically addressing addicted people differently than nonaddicted people, though only under strict limitations.

7. **A**

 The U.S. Supreme Court has considered "currently prevailing standards of decency" that "mark the progress of a maturing society" and as a result ruled against precedent set in prior cases. The *Roper v. Simmons* ruling went against precedent set in *Stanford v. Kentucky* and found that execution of juvenile offenders was a violation of the Eighth Amendment based on evidence that American society's opinion had evolved. The *Payne v. Tennessee* ruling did go against precedent set in *Booth v. Maryland*. However, this decision was not based on the evolution of America's opinion but rather the opinion of the court that the *Booth* decision had been "badly reasoned" and that stare decisis (common law concept that precedent is binding) was not an "inexorable command."

The *Ford v. Wainwright* decision cited a long-standing "ancestral legacy" in common law that stands against executing the insane.

8. **E**

    The U.S. Supreme Court did not opine about the substantive or procedural issues in the case. Rather, the focus was on whether Congress had the power to enact the federal statute that allowed for civil commitment of a sex offender after completion of his sentence. The Court had previously addressed issues of double jeopardy and equal protection as well as ex post facto and procedural standards in its opinions on state statutes, such as in *Kansas v. Hendricks*.

9. **D**

    The accused in a federal prosecution must prove incompetence by a "preponderance of the evidence" (more likely than not). *Cooper v. Oklahoma* held that an Oklahoma law proving a defendant's incompetence by "clear and convincing evidence" violates due process by allowing the state to put a defendant on trial who is more likely than not incompetent. The standard of "beyond a reasonable doubt" (used in criminal matters) is a higher standard than "clear and convincing evidence" and thus would make it even more likely that incompetent defendants are put on trial. "Without due cause" is not a recognized standard.

10. **D**

    In *People v. Patterson*, the New York Court of Appeals held that the state can place the burden of proving EED on the defendant without violating the defendant's constitutional due process protections. In EED cases, which are never civil in nature, the distress is not necessarily presumed and has nothing to do with insanity considerations.

11. **D**

    In *Miranda*, the suspect did indeed sign a confession in which he stated that he knew of his rights and that his statement may used against him—but only after he had been in custody for several hours. Therefore, the case was overturned not because he did not know his rights but because having been in custody for several hours, he might have felt coerced to confess even though the police may not have committed any particular misconduct. The remaining answers were not cited in this or any other case. Subsequent to *Miranda*, Congress passed a statute that appeared to return the standard for judging the admissibility of confessions to one of a "totality of circumstances." However, the *Miranda* decision survived several challenges, as recently as 2004, and the so-called Miranda warning remains a continuing requirement.

QUESTIONS ON CRIMINAL LAW AND INCARCERATION (185)

12. **D**

    The U.S. Supreme Court ruled in *Estelle v. Smith* that an inmate's Fifth Amendment right against self-incrimination and Sixth Amendment right to counsel had been violated when a psychiatrist conducted a competency to stand trial evaluation and later used information obtained at a sentencing hearing. The Court reasoned that his Fifth Amendment right was violated because he was not aware that he could refuse and that the information he provided could be used against him. The Court also reasoned that because there had been no notice to defense counsel, he did not have the opportunity to consult his counsel about whether or not he should participate.

13. **D**

    Prior to the *Hinckley* case, which prompted the Insanity Defense Reform Act of 1984, the burden of proof in federal courts was on the prosecution to prove a defendant's sanity beyond a reasonable double. The act shifted the burden of proof to the defendant to prove insanity by clear and convincing evidence.

14. **A**

    Drope v. Missouri held that competency should be considered at any time where sufficient doubt arises about a defendant's current competence in an effort to protect the defendant's right to a fair trial, which includes protection of his or her due process.

15. **C**

    This question has been addressed in the context of both prison-based treatment and postincarceration SVP programs. *McKune v. Lile*, 536 U.S. 24 (2002), concerns treatment during incarceration, with the finding that the Fifth Amendment is not violated by a prison clinical rehabilitation program with a legitimate penological objective if the consequences of refusal to participate are related to the program objective and are not significant hardships relative to the prison environment. *Allen v. Illinois*, 478 U.S. 364 (1986), found that due process did not require Fifth Amendment protections against self-incrimination in SVP acts.

16. **D**

    In *Montana v. Egelhoff*, the U.S. Supreme Court affirmed that state law was not required by due process to allow entry of evidence of voluntary intoxication in criminal cases. It based this decision on the fact that common law had not universally acknowledged voluntary intoxication as a mitigating factor. Citing examples such as hearsay, the Court went on to discuss how various classes of potential evidence are routinely excluded. The *Egelhoff* decision had nothing to do with the insanity defense, which is not available in all states.

17. **C**

The American Medical Association (AMA) states that physicians may not participate in executions. The AMA also states that testifying to competency to stand trial, testifying to relevant medical evidence during trial, or testifying to medical aspects of aggravating or mitigating circumstances during the penalty phase of a capital case does *not* constitute physician participation in an execution. The American Psychiatric Association (APA) Principles of Medical Ethics, with Annotations Especially Applicable to Psychiatry state that a psychiatrist should not participate in a legally authorized execution. Neither the APA nor the American Academy of Psychiatry and the Law (AAPL) prohibits psychiatrists from providing treatment to patients who are incompetent to be executed, although the AMA recommends that no psychiatrist treat an inmate solely for the purpose of restoring competence to be executed. The AAPL does not prohibit psychiatrists from conducting competency to be sentenced evaluations.

Please see the relevant ethical guidelines:
1AMA - http://www.ama-assn.org/ama/pub/physician-resources/medical-ethics/code-medical-ethics.page
APA - http://www.psych.org/practice/ethics
AAPL - http://www.aapl.org/ethics.htm

18. **A**

Voluntary and knowing. In *Miranda*, the Supreme Court determined that in order for a confession to be voluntary and knowing, the suspect who confessed had to have been apprised of his rights by the police. Informed consent is the standard for agreeing to medical procedures, established in, among other cases, *Natanson v. Kline*. Clear and convincing is a level of proof found in some civil cases where significant liberty interests are at stake, such as civil commitment and right to refuse treatment. Competence and intelligence are general terms that may be included in particular standards for decision making in civil and criminal matters.

19. **C**

Dusky v. U.S. first established that the test for competency to stand trial should be "whether he has sufficient present ability to consult with his lawyer with a reasonable degree of rational understanding -

and whether he has a rational as well as factual understanding of the proceedings against him." *Drope v. Missouri* held that competency to stand trial should be considered at any time during a trial where sufficient doubt as to the defendant's competency arises. *Jackson v. Indiana* held that indefinite commitment due to incompetency to stand trial was a violation of the Equal Protection Clause and Due Process Clauses of the Fourteenth Amendment. *Wilson v. U.S.* held that amnesia does not make defendants incompetent as long as they are able to assist their attorney, can testify on their own behalf, and can extrinsically reconstruct the evidence in light of their amnesia.

20. **E**
Ake v. Oklahoma found that a state's denial of an indigent, capital defendant's access to a psychiatric consultant if he or she is pursuing an insanity defense violates the Fourteenth Amendment's due process guarantee.

21. **C**
In *Ibn-Tamas v. U.S.*, the DC Court of Appeals reversed the trial court's decision in excluding expert testimony regarding the "battered wife syndrome." The court found that the expert's statements were beyond the knowledge of the ordinary jury and that the expert testimony likely had more probative value than prejudicial effect. The court did not opine on the legitimacy of the "battered wife syndrome" and in fact returned the case to the trial court to determine the legitimacy of the expert's credentials and of the syndrome in question. Both psychiatrists as well as psychologists can be expert in trauma-related reactions, and there is no blanket protection for retaliatory violence against one's abusers.

22. **D**
PTSD has the best acceptance in the *Diagnostic and Statistical Manual of Mental Disorders* and the best argument that the illness would preclude the ability to control his violence.

23. **C**
The Prison Litigation Reform Act (PLRA) of 1995 is a congressional statute designed to regulate and limit the number of cases filed by prisoners. In the 2011 Supreme Court case of *Brown v. Plata*, the State of California challenged the authority of a three-judge district court to order the reduction of the state prison population as a measure to improve deteriorating medical and mental health care for prisoners. The Supreme Court held that the lower court's decision was allowed under the PLRA.

24. **D**

A diminished capacity defense is not constitutionally required by due process (neither is a not guilty by reason of insanity plea) but is intimately concerned with a defendant's criminal state of mind and intent in the criminal act. Diminished capacity defenses originate from the defense but must be done so by a competent defendant. The benefit of using this defense is for mitigation, not acquittal (as in NGRI defenses).

25. **A**

SVP commitment proceedings have been found to be civil proceedings due to the goal of treatment rather than punishment. Therefore, the courts have ruled that due process requires that there be a finding of mental disorder, though the term can be defined in various ways, including by terms such as "mental illness" or "mental abnormality," and personality disorder may be considered. As with other forms of civil commitment hearings, the mental disorder in question must have a relationship with the individual's risk of committing sexual offenses.

26. **B**

Prison officials may be held liable for deliberate indifference only if they are aware of a "substantial risk of serious harm" and they "disregard that risk by failing to take reasonable measures to abate it." The 1994 Supreme Court case of *Farmer v. Brennan* involved a suit brought by a male-to-female transsexual who alleged a violation of her Eighth Amendment rights by prison officials after she was beaten and raped by another inmate in a federal penitentiary.

27. **E**

Ford v. Wainwright (1986) addressed the issue of a mentally ill person's competence to be executed and held that the Eighth Amendment prohibited the execution of the insane. *Atkins v. Virginia* (2002) found that execution of the mentally retarded was barred by the Eighth Amendment. *Roper v. Simmons* (2005) similarly found that it was unconstitutional to subject offenders who were under the age of 18 at the time of committing a capital offense to the death penalty. *Estelle v. Smith* (1981) dealt with the use of psychiatric testimony to predict future dangerousness. In *State v. Perry* (1992), the Louisiana Supreme Court addressed the question whether the state could give antipsychotic medication involuntarily to an incompetent death row inmate to make him competent to be executed.

QUESTIONS ON CRIMINAL LAW AND INCARCERATION (189)

28. **E**

    State v. Perry was a Louisiana Supreme Court case that determined that involuntary medication administered merely for the purpose of restoring competency for execution is an unjustified invasion of privacy and added a degrading indignity to the punishment that was cruel and excessive. In *Washington v. Harper*, the court considered whether a prisoner is entitled to a judicial hearing when seeking to refuse psychiatric medication and found that due process requires liberty interests to be balanced against the prisoner's medical interest and the state's interest in prison safety.

29. **B**

    In this case, Mr. Connelly had provided a full confession to murder while affected by command auditory hallucinations. The police taking the confession were not coercive in any way, but the confession was clearly not the result of a "rational intellect and free will." The Court held that police coercion was the determinative factor in deciding whether a confession should be suppressed. In the case, Miranda rights were clearly presented in a timely fashion. Illegal search and seizure are not relevant considerations to the appropriateness of a confession.

30. **B**

    Patients have substantive due process rights. These rights bar arbitrary wrongful governmental actions. Freedom from bodily restraint is at the core of the liberty protected by the Due Process Clause from arbitrary governmental action. The state must create procedural safeguards against unwarranted confinement. The defendant could argue that, in this case, a 5-year confinement prior to his first hearing is arbitrary.

31. **B**

    Vitek v. Jones was a 1980 U.S. Supreme Court case in which a Nebraska prisoner challenged the authority of the state to transfer him to a psychiatric hospital in violation of the Due Process Clause of the Fourteenth Amendment. The Court ruled that the transfer of a prisoner to a mental hospital has stigmatizing consequences beyond those imposed by incarceration and exposed Mr. Jones to treatment over his objection.

32. **E**

    The legal holding in *Connelly* pertains to the constitutional guarantee on due process of law, specifically that coercive police behavior is required to invalidate a confession. This protection is codified in the Fourteenth Amendment. The First Amendment protects freedom of speech, religion, and the press. The Second Amendment protects the right to bear arms. The Fourth Amendment prohibits unlawful search and seizure. The Eighth Amendment prohibits cruel and unusual punishment.

33. **B**

    In *Atkins v. Virginia*, the majority held that imposing the death penalty on the mentally retarded would not measurably contribute to the goals of retribution or deterrence. They reasoned that the deficiencies of mentally retarded offenders diminish their personal culpability such that the most extreme form of punishment is not warranted and that their cognitive and behavioral impairments made it unlikely that they would control their conduct based on knowledge of the possibility of the death penalty. The Court also considered that mentally retarded offenders are less able to meaningfully assist in their defense and as a result have an increased risk of wrongful execution. The Court also took into account the large number of states that prohibited the execution of the mentally retarded and polling data that showed consensus among Americans that executing the mentally retarded is wrong. Mental retardation in and of itself does not necessarily render an offender incompetent.

34. **D**

    The presence of mental disorder alone is not sufficient to find lack of control. The ruling in *Kansas v. Crane*, 534 U.S. 407 (2002), discussed the lack of "mathematical precision" possible in determining lack of control, in part because the distinction between "emotional" and "volitional" is not always clear. Complete lack of control over behavior is not necessary; proof of serious difficulty is adequate.

35. **B**

    Wilson v. U.S. a case heard in the U.S. Court of Appeals, DC Circuit, held that amnesia did not make a defendant incompetent if available ancillary information was available to construct knowledge of an event in order to mount a defense. It also held that such defendants should be able to follow the proceedings against them, discuss them rationally with their attorney, and testify on their own behalf.

36. **B**

    Under the Eighth Amendment, prison officials may be held liable if they are aware of a "substantial risk of serious harm" and they "disregard that risk by failing to take reasonable measures to abate it." The 1994 U.S. Supreme Court case of *Farmer v. Brennan* involved a suit brought by a male-to-female transsexual who alleged a violation of her Eighth Amendment rights by prison officials after she was beaten and raped by a male inmate in a federal penitentiary. The test applied to this case was that of "subjective recklessness."

37. **A**

In *Payne v. Tennessee*, the U.S. Supreme Court reconsidered its prior position in the *Booth* and *Gathers* decisions. The Court determined that victim impact statements should be allowed to aid a jury in understanding the "uniqueness" of the victim as an individual and in assessing the degree of harm caused by the crime, which is directly related to the defendant's moral culpability. The state should also be afforded the opportunity to rebut mitigating evidence presented by the defense at sentencing. It is possible that psychiatrists could be asked to testify about the psychological impact of the crime on the victim's family.

38. **B**

In this case the defendant presents with the cognitive difficulties required of M'Naghten. In the other scenarios the defendants' ability to control their actions may be in question, but they may all be aware of what they are doing or that what they are doing is wrong.

39. **E**

The "necessary and proper" clause is found in Article I of the Constitution, which specifies that Congress has the power "to make all law which shall be necessary and proper for carrying into execution the foregoing powers and all other powers vested by this Constitution." The First Amendment guarantees the right to free speech and assembly. The Fifth Amendment guarantees the right against self-incrimination. The Eighth Amendment prohibits cruel and unusual punishment. The Fourteenth Amendment guarantees due process and equal protection and is the amendment through which all the amendments are made obligatory on the states as well as the federal government.

40. **B**

An ALI jurisdiction states that a person is not responsible for criminal conduct if at the time of such conduct as a result of mental disease he lacks substantial capacity either to appreciate the wrongfulness of his conduct or to conform his conduct to the requirements of the law. Answer B comes closest to presenting a scenario in which the defendant was not able to appreciate the wrongfulness of his actions or to conform his conduct to the law.

41. E

In *Robinson v. California* (1968), the U.S. Supreme Court ruled that it was cruel and unusual punishment to arrest people for a status they could not control, if they had not performed any other antisocial or disorderly behavior. Possible intent to commit a crime in the undefined future is not in itself a prosecutable crime. All the other answer choices are taken directly from the text of the opinion as valid forms of state regulation. The Court ruled that states maintained broad powers to impose criminal sanctions against the unauthorized manufacture, prescription, sale, purchase, or possession of narcotics within their borders. It also ruled that it was not cruel and unusual to impose compulsory treatment for those addicted to narcotics—with periods of involuntary confinement as part of a treatment program—and penal sanctions for a failure to comply with established compulsory treatment procedures. Finally, the Court ruled that other strategies at the disposal of the states could include public health education and efforts to ameliorate the economic and social conditions under which drug abuse flourishes.

42. E

Answers (A) through (D) have all been raised in challenges to sexual offender commitment statutes. Double jeopardy and ex post facto lawmaking were raised by *In re Young and Cunningham*, 857 P.2d 989 (1993), and *Kansas v. Hendricks*, 521 U.S. 346 (1997). Due process issues were raised in *Specht v. Patterson*, 386 U.S. 605 (1967), *In re Young and Cunningham*, and *Kansas v. Hendricks*. The Fifth Amendment was addressed in *Allen v. Illinois*, 478 U.S. 364 (1986), and *McKune v. Lile*, 536 U.S. 24 (2002).

43. A

In supporting New York State's right to place the burden to prove aspects of EED on the defendant, the court of appeals differentiated the state's law from Maine's EED law, which had recently been struck down by the U.S. Supreme Court in *Mullaney v. Wilbur* (421 U.S. 684). The New York state law still required the state to prove all elements of the crime and so did not violate due process. The decision in *Patterson* was unrelated to its legislative history and has nothing to do with voluntary intoxication. EED is not based in the U.S. Constitution (being only available in certain states).

44. B

Mr. Powell was decidedly *not* convicted for the "status" of being an alcoholic, as this would have been in direct contradiction of *Robinson v. California.* He was in fact convicted for the "act" of being intoxicated in public; he was not alleged to have committed any other crime, including murder. The Court opinion briefly made reference to the debate regarding responsibility for criminal actions as it related to the insanity defense by mentioning two cases. In one, the U.S. Court of Appeals for the DC Circuit decided *Durham v. U.S.* (1954), adopting the "product test" to determine the validity of an insanity defense; it states that "an accused is not criminally responsible if his unlawful act was the product of mental disease or defect." The other, a historic English case, resulted in the M'Naghten rule, which stated in summary that insanity was a defense if the party was unable to tell right from wrong at the time of the crime. Other than using these cases as abstract legal analogies, the Court refused to define an insanity defense in constitutional terms and did not opine on their relationship to Mr. Powell's case.

45. **B**

    In *Sell v. U.S.* Dr. Sell was found incompetent to stand trial and while hospitalized refused antipsychotic medication. Forced medication was authorized, and Sell appealed. The U.S. Supreme Court ruled that the government is permitted to involuntarily administer antipsychotic medications to certain mentally ill defendants in order to render them competent to stand trial, but the Court outlined necessary procedures, which included that the treatment should be unlikely to have side effects that undermine fairness of a trial, that the recommended treatment should be the least intrusive and medically appropriate, and that the treatment should be necessary to further government trial-related interests.

46. **B**

    Indiana v. Edwards held that the Constitution permits states to insist upon counsel for those competent to stand trial under the standard set forth by *Dusky v. U.S.* but incompetent to conduct their own trial proceedings. The Court noted that *Dusky* alone was not sufficient and assumed representation within the standard itself. It also pointed to the variability in mental illness with regard to its course over time and the variability in the way it interferes with a defendant's function. Furthermore, permitting self-representation to a defendant who lacks the capacity to conduct his or her defense without counsel does not "affirm the dignity" of the defendant and does not "appear fair to all who observe them."

47. **E**

For years, the state of California failed to comply with court-ordered remedial efforts to improve the delivery of both medical and mental health care to its prisoners. In 2008, a three-judge district court combined two class action suits (one for medical care, one for mental health care) and ordered to have the prison population reduced to 137.5% of its designed capacity to rectify overcrowding in California prisons, which was determined to be a primary cause for the poor medical and mental health care.

48. **B**

This question is answered by *McKune v. Lile*, 536 U.S. 24 (2002). The prison program challenged by Lile required him to accept responsibility for the crime of conviction and detail prior sexual activities, including potential uncharged offenses, with refusal to participate leading to consequences of reduction in privileges and possible transfer to a higher-security unit. The Supreme Court decision allows for the program to be incentivized through prison privileges and holds that Fifth Amendment protections against self-incrimination do not prevent treatment programs from requiring participants to disclose sexual histories and prior behaviors. Availability of sex offender treatment during incarceration has been cited as an issue in legislative and mental health community discussions but has not been made a requirement by court decisions.

APPENDIX A

The Bill of Rights and Fourteenth Amendment, U.S. Constitution

Amendments I–X Ratified December 15, 1791; XIV ratified July 9, 1868
Source: www.archives.gov
The Preamble to the Bill of Rights
Congress of the United States
begun and held at the City of New-York, on
Wednesday the fourth of March, one thousand seven hundred and eighty nine.

THE Conventions of a number of the States, having at the time of their adopting the Constitution, expressed a desire, in order to prevent misconstruction or abuse of its powers, that further declaratory and restrictive clauses should be added: And as extending the ground of public confidence in the Government, will best ensure the beneficent ends of its institution.

RESOLVED by the Senate and House of Representatives of the United States of America, in Congress assembled, two thirds of both Houses concurring, that the following Articles be proposed to the Legislatures of the several States, as amendments to the Constitution of the United States, all, or any of which Articles, when ratified by three fourths of the said Legislatures, to be valid to all intents and purposes, as part of the said Constitution; viz.

ARTICLES in addition to, and Amendment of the Constitution of the United States of America, proposed by Congress, and ratified by the Legislatures of the several States, pursuant to the fifth Article of the original Constitution.

AMENDMENT I

Congress shall make no law respecting an establishment of religion, or prohibiting the free exercise thereof; or abridging the freedom of speech, or of the press; or the right of the people peaceably to assemble, and to petition the Government for a redress of grievances.

AMENDMENT II

A well regulated Militia, being necessary to the security of a free State, the right of the people to keep and bear Arms, shall not be infringed.

AMENDMENT III

No Soldier shall, in time of peace be quartered in any house, without the consent of the Owner, nor in time of war, but in a manner to be prescribed by law.

AMENDMENT IV

The right of the people to be secure in their persons, houses, papers, and effects, against unreasonable searches and seizures, shall not be violated, and no Warrants shall issue, but upon probable cause, supported by Oath or affirmation, and particularly describing the place to be searched, and the persons or things to be seized.

AMENDMENT V

No person shall be held to answer for a capital, or otherwise infamous crime, unless on a presentment or indictment of a Grand Jury, except in cases arising in the land or naval forces, or in the Militia, when in actual service in time of War or public danger; nor shall any person be subject for the same offence to be twice put in jeopardy of life or limb; nor shall be compelled in any criminal case to be a witness against himself, nor be deprived of life, liberty, or property, without due process of law; nor shall private property be taken for public use, without just compensation.

AMENDMENT VI

In all criminal prosecutions, the accused shall enjoy the right to a speedy and public trial, by an impartial jury of the State and district wherein the crime shall have been committed, which district shall have been previously ascertained by law, and to be informed of the nature and cause of the accusation; to be confronted with the witnesses against him; to have compulsory process for obtaining witnesses in his favor, and to have the Assistance of Counsel for his defence.

AMENDMENT VII

In Suits at common law, where the value in controversy shall exceed twenty dollars, the right of trial by jury shall be preserved, and no fact tried by a jury, shall be otherwise re-examined in any Court of the United States, than according to the rules of the common law.

AMENDMENT VIII

Excessive bail shall not be required, nor excessive fines imposed, nor cruel and unusual punishments inflicted.

AMENDMENT IX

The enumeration in the Constitution, of certain rights, shall not be construed to deny or disparage others retained by the people.

AMENDMENT X

The powers not delegated to the United States by the Constitution, nor prohibited by it to the States, are reserved to the States respectively, or to the people.

AMENDMENT XIV

Section 1

All persons born or naturalized in the United States, and subject to the jurisdiction thereof, are citizens of the United States and of the State wherein they reside. No State shall make or enforce any law which shall abridge the privileges or immunities of citizens of the United States; nor shall any State deprive any person of life, liberty, or property, without due process of law; nor deny to any person within its jurisdiction the equal protection of the laws.

Section 2

Representatives shall be apportioned among the several States according to their respective numbers, counting the whole number of persons in each State, excluding Indians not taxed. But when the right to vote at any election for the choice of electors for President and Vice-President of the United States, Representatives in Congress, the Executive and Judicial officers of a State, or the members of the Legislature thereof, is denied to any of the male inhabitants of such State, being twenty-one years of age,* and citizens of the United States, or in any way abridged, except for participation in rebellion, or other crime, the basis of representation therein shall be reduced in the proportion which the number of such male citizens shall bear to the whole number of male citizens twenty-one years of age in such State.

Section 3

No person shall be a Senator or Representative in Congress, or elector of President and Vice-President, or hold any office, civil or military, under the United States, or under any State, who, having previously taken an oath, as a member of Congress, or as an officer of the United States, or as a member of any State legislature, or as an executive or judicial officer of any State, to support the Constitution of the United States, shall have engaged in insurrection or rebellion against the same, or given aid or comfort to the enemies thereof. But Congress may by a vote of two-thirds of each House, remove such disability.

Section 4

The validity of the public debt of the United States, authorized by law, including debts incurred for payment of pensions and bounties for services in suppressing insurrection or rebellion, shall not be questioned. But neither the United States nor any State shall assume or pay any debt or obligation incurred in aid of insurrection or rebellion against the United States, or any claim for the loss or emancipation of any slave; but all such debts, obligations and claims shall be held illegal and void.

Section 5

The Congress shall have the power to enforce, by appropriate legislation, the provisions of this article.

APPENDIX B

General Path to the U.S. Supreme Court

State:
   Local trial court → Appellate court → State supreme court → U.S. Supreme Court

Federal:
   District court → U.S. Court of Appeals → U.S. Supreme Court

APPENDIX C

Geographic Boundaries of the U.S. and DC Circuit Courts of Appeal

Geographic Boundaries
of United States Courts of Appeals and United States District Courts

Reproduced from http://www.uscourts.gov/uscourts/images/CircuitMap.pdf

INDEX

Abuse of children. See Child abuse
Abuse of discretion standard for expert testimony, 23–24, 33
ADA. See Americans with Disabilities Act (ADA)
ADA Amendments Act of 2008, 124
Admissibility of confessions, 186
Adolescents. See Children and adolescents
Alcoholism, public intoxication resulting from as crime, 134, 192–193
Alford pleas, 132, 181–182
American Academy of Psychiatry and the Law, xix, 173, 186
American Board of Forensic Psychiatry, xx
American Board of Medical Specialties, xx
American Board of Psychiatry and Neurology, xx–xxii, 63, 95
American Law Institute (ALI), 148, 175, 179, 187, 191
American Medical Association, 60, 65, 117, 122, 173–174, 186
American Psychiatric Association, 38, 117, 122, 173, 186
Americans with Disabilities Act (ADA)
  generally, 95, 118, 120, 124
  continued hospitalization of mentally ill persons beyond clinical need as discrimination, 99–100
  HIV status as disability under, 98
  major life activities, disability affecting, 98, 100–101
  prisoners, applicability to, 99, 102
  sovereign immunity and, 102
  specific work-related tasks, disability limited to not covered by ADA, 100–101, 126
  telecommunications and, 124

Amnesia, effect on competency to stand trial, 136, 190
Antipsychotic medication
  civilly committed persons, refusal by, 56–57, 67–68
  competency to stand trial, administration of antipsychotic medication to prisoners to restore, 155, 193
  consent by guardians to involuntary administration of, 55–56, 66
  death penalty, administration to restore competency to be executed, 160, 189
  determination that antipsychotic medication for prisoners medically appropriate and least intrusive option required, 153–154
  hearings on administration to prisoners, 152–153
  liability for failure to obtain informed consent, 13, 37–38
  patient noncompliance, duty to protect third parties from consequences of, 17
Arizona Penal Code, 149
Attorney, right to
  involuntary commitment, 68
  pretrial psychiatric evaluations, death penalty proceedings, 185
Autonomy, civil commitment and, 67

Battered child syndrome, liability for failure to diagnose, 73–74
Battered woman syndrome, diminished capacity and, 142, 187
Bazelon, David, 51, 146
Best interests of child standard, child custody, 76–77, 91, 93–94

(205)

Billing fraud, subpoena of records for, 7
Bill of Rights, 195–197
Blackmun, Harry, 91
Bodily restraint, freedom from, 52–53, 69
Burden of proof
  child custody, best interests of child standard, 76–77, 91, 93–94
  civil commitment, clear and convincing evidence standard, 46–47, 66
  competency to stand trial, preponderance of evidence standard, 139–140, 184
  extreme emotional disturbance, 141, 184, 192
  insanity defense, 185
  termination of parental rights, preponderance of evidence standard, 77, 89–93
Bush, George H.W., 124
Bush, George W., 124

California Penal Code, 74
Capacity, diminished. *See* Diminished capacity
Capital punishment. *See* Death penalty
Catheterization during school hours for students with spina bifida, 82–83
Child abuse, 73–75
  battered child syndrome, liability for failure to diagnose, 73–74
  constitutional obligation of state to protect children from abuse by private citizens, 75, 93
  physicians, reporting requirements, 92–93
  psychotherapist-patient privilege, applicability to reporting requirements, 74, 90
Child custody, best interests of child standard, 76–77, 91, 93–94
Children and adolescents, 71–94
  generally, 71
  child abuse, 73–75 (*See also* Child abuse)
  child custody, best interests of child standard, 76–77, 91, 93–94
  civil commitment, adversarial hearing requirement, 47, 66–67

death penalty, 161–162, 182
disabled students, 81–83 (*See also* Disabled students)
EAHCA, 81–83 (*See also* Education for All Handicapped Children Act (EAHCA))
juvenile rights, 78–80 (*See also* Juvenile rights)
questions, 84–94
termination of parental rights, preponderance of evidence standard, 77, 89–93
Circuit Courts of Appeals, geographic boundaries of, 204
Civil commitment, 43–47
  generally, 64
  antipsychotic medication, refusal of, 56–57, 67–68
  autonomy and, 67
  clear and convincing evidence standard, 46–47, 66
  due process rights, 45
  least restrictive alternatives, involuntary commitment when available, 43–44, 64
  minimally adequate standards for psychiatric treatment, 52, 65
  minors, adversarial hearing requirement, 47, 66–67
  non-dangerous mentally ill persons, involuntary commitment, 45–46
  police power and, 67
  release from prison, jury determination required for civil commitment, 44, 69
  right to refuse treatment, 57–58
  sex offenders, civil commitment beyond scheduled release date, 168, 184, 191
  sexually violent predator statute, civil commitment procedure not violating constitutional protections, 165–166, 192
Civil Rights Act of 1964
  generally, 119
  definition of hostile work environment sexual harassment, 125, 127
  injury to psychological well-being not required for hostile environment sexual harassment, 113

quid pro quo linkage not required for sexual harassment, 112–113
same-sex sexual harassment under, 114
Civil Rights of Institutionalized Persons Act of 1980, 41
Clear and convincing evidence standard
civil commitment, 46–47, 66
removal of life-sustaining treatment, 48–49, 64, 68
Clinical experience, expert testimony and, 38
Cognitive unawareness of right and wrong, insanity defense, 144–145, 191
Commitment
civil commitment (*See* Civil commitment)
involuntary commitment (*See* Involuntary commitment)
voluntary commitment, incompetent persons unable to consent to, 14
Communications Act of 1934, 124
Competency to stand trial, 135–140
generally, 185–187
amnesia, effect of, 136, 190
antipsychotic medication, administration to prisoners to restore, 155, 193
basic knowledge of charges, sufficiency of, 135–136
indefinite commitment of persons found incompetent, 136–137
insanity defense, waiver of, 146–147
interruption of criminal proceedings where defendant appears to lack, 137–138
preponderance of evidence standard, 139–140, 184
self-representation, standard for compared, 140, 193
waiver of constitutional rights, standard for compared, 138–139
Compulsive gambling not establishing insanity defense, 147–148
Confessions
admissibility of, 186
coercive police activity and lack of voluntariness, 132–133, 189–190
Miranda rights, 131, 184, 186, 189

Confidentiality and privilege, 3–9
billing fraud, subpoena of records for, 7
child abuse reporting, applicability of privilege to, 74, 90
dangerous persons, applicability of privilege to records, 8
federal courts, privilege in, 8–9
grand jury subpoena, contempt for refusal to respond to, 5–6
group therapy, privilege extending to, 6–7, 38
mandatory reporting requirements and, 34, 37
privilege defined, 34–35
publication of information, 4
state, collection of personal information by, 5
waiver of privilege, 3–4
Consent. *See* Informed consent
Constitution. *See specific Clause or Amendment*
Contempt, refusal to respond to grand jury subpoena, 5–6
Counsel, right to
involuntary commitment, 68
pretrial psychiatric evaluations, death penalty proceedings, 185
Courts of Appeals, geographic boundaries of, 204
Criminal law, 129–194
generally, 129
competency to stand trial, 135–140 (*See also* Competency to stand trial)
criminal procedure, 131–134 (*See also* Criminal procedure)
death penalty, 157–162 (*See also* Death penalty)
diminished capacity, 141–143 (*See also* Diminished capacity)
insanity defense, 144–150 (*See also* Insanity defense)
prisoners' rights, 151–156 (*See also* Prisoners' rights)
questions, 169–194
self-representation, standard for, 140, 193
sex offenders, 163–168 (*See also* Sex offenders)
waiver of constitutional rights, standard for, 138–139

Criminal procedure, 131–134
  confessions (*See* Confessions)
  drug addiction status as crime, 133, 183, 192
  guilty pleas, 132, 181–182
  informing suspects of rights, 131
  public intoxication resulting from alcoholism as crime, 134, 192–193

Damages, punitive
  health insurance, companies, recovery from, 124
  malpractice insurance coverage of, 106
Dangerous persons
  insanity acquitees, dangerousness and mental illness required for continued hospitalization, 148–149
  records, applicability of privilege to, 8
  sex offenders, proof of inability to control behavior not required, 167
  third parties, duty to protect from, 15–16, 33, 36, 38–39
Daubert test, 23–24, 34–35, 38
Death, right to. *See* Right to die
Death penalty, 157–162
  admissibility of evidence from pretrial psychiatric evaluations, 157
  competency to be executed, administration of antipsychotic medication to restore, 160, 189
  evolving standards of decency and, 183–184
  indigent persons, access to pretrial psychiatric evaluations, 158, 187
  insane persons, 158–159, 188
  mentally ill persons, 90
  mentally retarded persons, 160–161, 182, 190
  minors, 161–162, 182
  physicians and, 186
  psychotherapists and, 186
  "rational understanding" and "factual awareness" required for competency to be executed, 162
  victim impact statements, admissibility during sentencing, 159, 191
Delaware Psychiatric Association, 19

Deliberate indifference required to support prisoners' claims for denial of right to treatment, 151–152, 154–155, 188, 190–191
Delinquency. *See* Juvenile rights
Diagnostic and Statistical Manual of Mental Disorders, 27, 34, 187
Diminished capacity, 141–143
  generally, 182, 188
  battered woman syndrome and, 142, 187
  due process, exclusion of evidence of voluntary intoxication and, 143
  extreme emotional disturbance, burden of proof, 141, 184, 192
  murder charge, effect of voluntary intoxication on, 142–143
  prejudicial impact, effect of, 142, 187
Disabled persons, 97–102
  continued hospitalization of mentally ill persons beyond clinical need as discrimination, 99–100
  durable power of attorney for mentally ill persons, 101, 122–123
  HIV status as disability, 98
  major life activities, disability affecting, 98, 100–101
  prisoners, applicability of ADA to, 99, 102
  specific work-related tasks, disability limited to not covered by ADA, 100–101, 126
  timely community care for, 121
  workers' compensation, compensability for emotional injuries under, 97–98, 124–125
Disabled students, 81–83
  hemodialysis for, 90–91
  Individualized Education Plans, 81–82
  spina bifida, catheterization during school hours for students with, 82–83
  standard of education required under EAHCA, 81–82, 89, 91
Doctors. *See* Physicians
Double jeopardy, sexually violent predator statutes not violating prohibition against, 164–166, 192
Drugs
  addiction status as crime, 133, 183, 192

antipsychotic medication (*See*
    Antipsychotic medication)
prescription drugs, personal
    information collected by state, 5
Due Process Clause
    child abuse, constitutional obligation
        of state to protect against, 75, 93
    civil commitment and, 45
    competency to stand trial,
        preponderance of evidence
        standard, 139–140
    confessions, coercive police activity
        and lack of voluntariness, 132–133,
        189–190
    confinement of insanity acquitees for
        longer duration than imprisonment
        for conviction, 147
    expert testimony under, 21
    extreme emotional disturbance,
        burden of proof, 184, 192
    hearings on administration of
        antipsychotic medication to
        prisoners, 152–153
    indigent persons, access to
        pretrial psychiatric evaluations
        in death penalty proceedings,
        158, 187
    juvenile delinquents, procedural due
        process rights coextensive with
        rights of adults, 79
    physician-assisted suicide, right to,
        49, 67
    prisoners, procedural protections
        regarding involuntary commitment
        of, 152, 189
    right to treatment for hospitalized
        insanity acquitees, 51–52, 65
    voluntary intoxication, effect of
        exclusion of evidence of, 143
Durable power of attorney for mentally
    ill persons, 101, 122–123
Durham rule, 145
Duty to protect, 15–19
    generally, 32, 38
    in absence of specific threat, 17–18
    dangerous persons, duty to protect
        third parties from, 15–16, 33, 36,
        38–39
    foreseeable but unidentified third
        parties, 16–17

former patients, duty to protect public
    from, 18–19, 35–36
patient noncompliance with
    medication, duty to protect third
    parties from consequences of, 17

Education for All Handicapped Children
    Act (EAHCA), 81–83
    generally, 71, 84
    spina bifida, catheterization during
        school hours for students with,
        82–83
    standard of education required under,
        81–82, 89, 91
EED. *See* Extreme emotional disturbance,
    burden of proof
Eighth Amendment
    generally, 190
    bodily restraint, freedom from, 52–53
    competency to stand trial, indefinite
        commitment of persons found
        lacking, 136–137
    drug addiction status as crime, 133
    habilation, 52–53
    juvenile delinquents, sentencing to life
        without parole, 79–80, 90, 93–94
    mentally retarded persons, death
        penalty and, 161
    minors, death penalty and, 161
    overcrowding of prisons, 156
    prisoners, applicability of ADA to, 102
    public intoxication resulting from
        alcoholism as crime, 134
    right to treatment, deliberate
        indifference required to support
        prisoner's claim for denial of, 151,
        188, 190–191
    safe conditions, 52–53
    text of, 197
    victim impact statements,
        admissibility during sentencing in
        death penalty proceedings, 159
Eleventh Amendment, ADA and, 102
Emotional harm, 103–104
    generally, 126
    actual physical injury not present,
        liability for negligence, 103–104
    damages for, 125
    foreseeability standard, 104, 124
    negligent infliction of, 122, 126

Emotional harm (*Cont.*)
  sex with patients, caused by, 127
  workers' compensation, compensability under, 97–98, 124–125
  zone of danger, 123
Employee benefit plans under ERISA, 125, 127
Employee Retirement Income Security Act of 1974 (ERISA)
  generally, 116, 119, 121–122
  employee benefit plans under, 125, 127
  health insurance surcharges, preemption of, 109
  HMOs, preemption of state malpractice claims against, 109–110
  malpractice claim preemption generally, 121
  utilization review, preemption of state malpractice claims, 108, 110–111
Engineers, expert testimony by, 24
Equal Employment Opportunity Commission, 113
Equal Protection Clause
  bodily restraint, freedom from, 52–53
  habilitation, 52–53
  insanity acquitees, dangerousness and mental illness required for continued hospitalization, 149
  physician-assisted suicide, right to, 49–50, 67
  safe conditions, 52–53
ERISA. *See* Employee Retirement Income Security Act of 1974 (ERISA)
Evolving standards of decency, death penalty and, 183–184
Experimental psychosurgery, involuntary commitment precluding necessity of informed consent, 11–12, 33
Expert testimony, 20–24
  abuse of discretion standard, 23–24, 33
  clinical experience and, 38
  Daubert test, 23–24, 34–35, 38
  engineers, testimony by, 24
  Frye test, 20, 23, 32–34
  general acceptance test, 20, 34
  hypnotically refreshed testimony, 21–22, 32, 34–37

  insanity defense, 145–146
  nonscientific testimony, 24
  relevancy and reliable foundation test, 23
  scientific community, admissibility of evidence not accepted by, 20
Ex post facto laws, sexually violent predator statutes not violating prohibition against, 164–166, 192
Extreme emotional disturbance, burden of proof, 141, 184, 192

"Factual awareness" required for competency to be executed, 162
Federal Comprehensive Alcohol Abuse and Alcoholism Prevention, Treatment and Rehabilitation Act Amendments of 1974, 6–7, 30, 37
Federal courts, privilege in, 8–9
Federal Rules of Evidence
  expert testimony under, 23, 27, 34
  hypnotically refreshed testimony, 35
  privilege in federal courts, 9
Federal Tort Claims Act, duty to protect under, 16, 18
Fifth Amendment
  admissibility of evidence from pretrial psychiatric evaluations, death penalty proceedings, 157
  competency to stand trial, effect of amnesia on, 136
  expert testimony under, 22
  guilty pleas, 132, 181–182
  incentives to participate in sexual abuse treatment program not violating self-incrimination privilege, 166–167, 185, 194
  informing suspects of rights, 131
  pretrial psychiatric evaluations, death penalty proceedings, self-incrimination privilege and, 185
  sex offenders, self-incrimination privilege and, 164, 166–167, 185
  text of, 196
First Amendment
  generally, 189–190
  text of, 196
Foreseeability
  absence of specific threat, duty to protect, 17–18

emotional harm, 104, 124
foreseeable but unidentified third parties, duty to protect, 16–17
Former patients, duty to protect public from, 18–19, 35–36
Fourteenth Amendment
  bodily restraint, freedom from, 52–53
  child abuse, constitutional obligation of state to protect against, 75, 93
  civil commitment under, 46
  competency to stand trial, preponderance of evidence standard, 139–140
  confessions, coercive police activity and lack of voluntariness, 132–133, 189–190
  confinement of insanity acquitees for longer duration than imprisonment for conviction, 147
  determination that antipsychotic medication for prisoners medically appropriate and least intrusive option required, 153–154
  expert testimony under, 21–22
  habilitation, 52–53
  hearings on administration of antipsychotic medication to prisoners, 152–153
  indigent persons, access to pretrial psychiatric evaluations in death penalty proceedings, 158, 187
  juvenile delinquents, procedural due process rights coextensive with rights of adults, 79
  minors, death penalty and, 161
  physician-assisted suicide, right to, 49–50, 67
  prisoners, applicability of ADA to, 102
  procedural protections regarding involuntary commitment of prisoners, 152, 189
  right to treatment for hospitalized insanity acquitees, 51–52, 65
  safe conditions, 52–53
  self-incrimination privilege, sex offenders and, 164
  sex offenders, sentencing under different statute precluded without hearing, 163
  text of, 198–199

voluntary intoxication, effect of exclusion of evidence of, 143
waiver of constitutional rights, standard for, 139
Fourth Amendment
  generally, 190
  text of, 196
Fraud, subpoena of records for, 7
Frye test, 20, 23, 32–34

Gambling, compulsive, not establishing insanity defense, 147–148
General acceptance test for expert testimony, 20, 34
Geographic boundaries of Courts of Appeals, 204
Georgia Department of Resources, 99
Grand jury subpoena, contempt for refusal to respond to, 5–6
Group therapy, privilege extending to, 6–7, 38
Guardians
  antipsychotic medication, consent to involuntary administration of, 55–56, 66
  substituted judgment standard, right to refuse treatment and, 55, 64, 68–69
Guilty pleas, 132, 181–182

Habilitation, right to, 52–53, 69
Handicapped persons. *See* Disabled persons
Handicapped students. *See* Disabled students
Harassment, sexual. *See* Sexual harassment
Health insurance, 105–111
  cost containment system affecting physician's medical judgment, liability for, 106–107
  HMOs, preemption of state malpractice claims against, 109–110
  liability for decisions in utilization review, 107–108
  physicians and, 121, 126
  punitive damages recovered from, 124
  surcharges, ERISA preemption of, 109
  utilization review, preemption of state malpractice claims, 108, 110–111

Health Insurance Portability and
    Accountability Act of 1996, 27, 34
Health maintenance organizations
    (HMOs), ERISA preemption of
    state malpractice claims against,
    109–110
Hearings
    antipsychotic medication,
        administration to prisoners,
        152–153
    civil commitment of children and
        adolescents, adversarial hearing
        requirement, 47, 66–67
    insanity acquitees, involuntary
        commitment of, 189
    sex offenders, sentencing under
        different statute precluded without
        hearing, 163–164
HIV status as disability, 98
Hostile work environment sexual
    harassment
    defined, 125, 127
    injury to psychological well-being not
        required, 113
    quid pro quo linkage not required,
        112–113
Hypnotically refreshed testimony,
    21–22, 32, 34–37

IDEA (Individuals with Disabilities
    Education Act), 84
Illinois Sexually Dangerous Persons Act,
    164
Imminent danger of death, effect on
    religious objections to treatment,
    54–55, 65
Incarceration. *See* Prisoners' rights
Incompetent persons unable to consent
    to voluntary commitment, 14, 36
Indigent persons, access to pretrial
    psychiatric evaluations in death
    penalty proceedings, 158, 187
Individualized Education Plans, 81–82
Individuals with Disabilities Education
    Act (IDEA), 84
Informed consent, 10–14
    generally, 37
    antipsychotic medication, liability for
        failure to obtain informed consent,
        13, 37–38
    experimental psychosurgery,
        involuntary commitment
        precluding necessity of informed
        consent, 11–12, 33
    incompetent persons unable to
        consent to voluntary commitment,
        14, 36
    medical tests, liability for
        nondisclosure of consequences of
        refusal, 12–13, 39
    physician care, required for, 10
    severe but rare inherent risks of
        medical procedures, liability for
        nondisclosure, 11
Insane persons, death penalty for,
    158–159, 188
Insanity defense, 144–150
    ALI rule, 148, 187, 191
    burden of proof, 185
    cognitive unawareness of right and
        wrong, 144–145, 191
    competency to waive, 146–147
    compulsive gambling not establishing,
        147–148
    dangerousness and mental
        illness required for continued
        hospitalization, 148–149
    Durham rule, 145
    expert testimony on, 145–146
    hearing required for involuntary
        commitment of acquitees, 189
    involuntary commitment of
        acquitees for longer duration than
        imprisonment for conviction, 147
    M'Naghten rule, 144–145, 191
    Mott rule, 149–150
    "product of mental disease or defect"
        test, 145
    right to treatment for hospitalized
        acquitees, 51–52, 65
    volitional element of, 149–150, 190
Insanity Defense Reform Act of 1984,
    172, 185
Institutional treatment guidelines, 41–69
    generally, 41
    civil commitment, 43–47 (*See also*
        Civil commitment)
    questions, 59–69
    right to die, 48–50 (*See also* Right
        to die)

right to refuse treatment, 54–58
(*See also* Right to refuse treatment)
right to treatment, 51–53 (*See also*
Right to treatment)
Insurance
health insurance (*See* Health insurance)
malpractice insurance (*See* Malpractice)
Intoxication
due process, exclusion of evidence of
voluntary intoxication and, 143,
185–186
murder charge, effect on, 142–143
public intoxication resulting from
alcoholism as crime, 134, 192–193
Involuntary commitment
competency to stand trial, indefinite
commitment of persons found
lacking, 136–137
confinement of insanity acquitees for
longer duration than imprisonment
for conviction, 147
continued hospitalization of mentally
ill persons beyond clinical need as
discrimination, 99–100
dangerousness and mental
illness required for continued
hospitalization of insanity
acquitees, 148–149
experimental psychosurgery, necessity
of informed consent precluded,
11–12, 33
insanity acquitees, hearing required,
189
least restrictive alternatives, when
available, 43–44, 64
non-dangerous mentally ill persons,
45–46
prisoners, procedural protections for,
152, 189
right to counsel, 68

Jurisdiction, right to treatment, 65
Juvenile rights, 78–80
generally, 86, 92
court proceedings, 92
life without parole, sentencing to,
79–80, 90, 93–94
procedural due process rights
coextensive with rights of adults,
78–79

Kansas Sexually Violent Predator Act,
165–167

Least restrictive alternatives,
involuntary commitment when
available, 43–44, 64

Major life activities, disabilities affecting,
98, 100–101
Malpractice
generally, 127
antipsychotic medication, liability for
failure to obtain informed consent,
13, 37–38
ERISA preemption of state malpractice
claims, 108–111, 121
insurance coverage of sex between
physician and patient, 105–106,
122
punitive damages, insurance coverage
of, 106
severe but rare inherent risks of
medical procedures, liability for
nondisclosure, 11
sex between psychotherapist and
patient as, 115
Massachusetts Department of Mental
Health, 57
Medicaid, 109
Medicaid False Claims Act, 7
Medical tests, liability for nondisclosure of
consequences of refusal, 12–13, 39
Medicare, 109
Mental health practice guidelines, 1–39
generally, 1
confidentiality, 3–9 (*See also*
Confidentiality and privilege)
duty to protect, 15–19 (*See also* Duty
to protect)
expert testimony, 20–24 (*See also*
Expert testimony)
informed consent, 10–14 (*See also*
Informed consent)
privilege, 3–9 (*See also* Confidentiality
and privilege)
questions, 25–39
Mentally ill persons
continued hospitalization beyond
clinical need as discrimination,
99–100

Mentally ill persons (*Cont.*)
  death penalty for, 90
  durable power of attorney for, 101, 122–123
  insane persons, death penalty for, 158–159, 188
  insanity acquitees, dangerousness and mental illness required for continued hospitalization, 148–149
  mentally retarded persons, death penalty for, 160–161, 182, 190
  minimally adequate standards for psychiatric treatment, 52, 65
  non-dangerous mentally ill persons, involuntary commitment, 45–46
  overcrowding of prisons and, 156, 187, 194
  right to refuse treatment, 183
Mentally retarded persons
  death penalty, 160–161, 182, 190
  minimally adequate standards for psychiatric treatment, 52, 65
Michigan Workman's Compensation Appeals Board, 97
Minimally adequate standards for psychiatric treatment, 52, 65
Minors. *See* Children and adolescents
Miranda rights, 131, 184, 186, 189
M'Naghten rule, 144–145, 191
Mott rule, 149–150

Necessary and Proper Clause, 168, 179, 191
Negligent infliction of emotional harm, 122, 126
New York
  Controlled Substances Act, 5
  Department of Correction, 44
  Department of Mental Hygiene, 44
  Family Court Act, 93
  Public Health Law, 109
New York University, xx
NGRI. *See* Insanity defense
Ninth Amendment, 197
Nondisclosure
  medical tests, liability for nondisclosure of consequences of refusal, 12–13, 39
  severe but rare inherent risks of medical procedures, liability for nondisclosure, 11
Nonscientific expert testimony, 24
Not guilty by reason of insanity. *See* Insanity defense

Overcrowding of prisons, 156, 187, 194

Parental rights, termination of, preponderance of evidence standard, 77, 89–93
Paternalism, 35
Pennsylvania Department of Corrections, 99
Permanent retrograde amnesia, effect on competency to stand trial, 136, 190
Personal information collected by state, 5
Physician-assisted suicide
  generally, 65–67
  due process right to, 49
  equal protection right to, 49–50
Physicians
  battered child syndrome, liability for failure to diagnose, 73–74
  child abuse reporting requirements, 92–93
  cost containment system affecting physician's medical judgment, liability of health insurance for, 106–107
  death penalty and, 186
  health insurance and, 121, 126
  informed consent, requirement for physician care, 10
  malpractice (*See* Malpractice)
  sex with patients and, 105–106, 122
Police power, civil commitment and, 67
Post-traumatic stress disorder, 187
Preemption under ERISA
  generally, 119
  employee benefit plans, 125
  health insurance surcharges, 109
  HMOs, state malpractice claims against, 109–110
  malpractice claim preemption generally, 121
  utilization review, state malpractice claims, 108, 110–111

Preponderance of evidence standard
  competency to stand trial, 139–140, 184
  termination of parental rights, 77, 89–93
Prescription drugs, personal information collected by state, 5
Pretrial psychiatric evaluations, death penalty
  admissibility of evidence from, 157
  indigent persons, access by, 158, 187
  right to counsel and, 185
  self-incrimination privilege and, 185
Prisoners' rights, 151–156
  ADA, applicability of, 99, 102
  competency to stand trial, administration of antipsychotic medication to restore, 155, 193
  determination that antipsychotic medication medically appropriate and least intrusive option required, 153–154
  hearings on administration of antipsychotic medication, 152–153
  involuntary commitment, procedural protections regarding, 152, 189
  overcrowding and, 156, 187, 194
  release from prison, jury determination required for civil commitment, 44, 69
  right to treatment, deliberate indifference required to support claim for denial of, 151–152, 154–155, 188, 190–191
Prison Litigation Reform Act of 1995, 156, 187
Privilege. *See* Confidentiality and privilege
Procedural due process rights of juvenile delinquents coextensive with rights of adults, 78–79
Proof, burden of. *See* Burden of proof
Pro se representation, standard for, 140, 193
Protect, duty to. *See* Duty to protect
Psychiatric evaluations. *See* Pretrial psychiatric evaluations, death penalty
Psychotherapists
  death penalty and, 186

psychotherapist-patient privilege (*See* Confidentiality and privilege)
  sex with patients and, 115, 122
Publication of information, confidentiality and, 4
Punitive damages
  health insurance, companies, recovery from, 124
  malpractice insurance coverage of, 106

Quid pro quo linkage not required for sexual harassment, 112–113

"Rational understanding" required for competency to be executed, 162
Refusal of treatment, right to. *See* Right to refuse treatment
Relevancy and reliable foundation test for expert testimony, 23
Religious objections to treatment, effect of imminent danger of death, 54–55, 65
Removal of life-sustaining treatment, clear and convincing evidence standard, 48–49, 64, 68
Right to counsel
  involuntary commitment, 68
  pretrial psychiatric evaluations, death penalty proceedings, 185
Right to die, 48–50
  due process right to physician-assisted suicide, 49
  equal protection right to physician-assisted suicide, 49–50
  physician-assisted suicide generally, 65–67
  removal of life-sustaining treatment, clear and convincing evidence standard, 48–49, 64, 68
Right to refuse treatment, 54–58
  antipsychotic medication, refusal by civilly committed persons, 56–57, 67–68
  civilly committed persons, refusal by, 57–58
  consent by guardians to involuntary administration of antipsychotic medication, 55–56, 66
  mentally ill persons, 183

Right to refuse treatment (*Cont.*)
  religious objections, effect of imminent danger of death, 54–55, 65
  substituted judgment standard, guardians and, 55, 64, 68–69
Right to treatment, 51–53
  bodily restraint, freedom from, 52–53, 69
  habilitation, 52–53, 69
  insanity defense, right to treatment for hospitalized acquitees, 51–52, 65
  jurisdiction, 65
  minimally adequate standards for psychiatric treatment, 52, 65
  prisoners, deliberate indifference required to support claim for denial of, 151–152, 154–155, 188, 190–191
  safe conditions, 52–53, 69

Safe conditions, right to, 52–53, 69
Same-sex sexual harassment, 114
Scientific community, admissibility of evidence not accepted by, 20
Second Amendment
  generally, 190
  text of, 196
Self-incrimination privilege
  civil proceedings involving sex offenders, inapplicable to, 164
  incentives for sex offenders to participate in sexual abuse treatment program not violating, 166–167, 185, 194
  pretrial psychiatric evaluations, death penalty proceedings, 185
Self-representation, standard for, 140, 193
Sentencing
  death penalty, 157–162 (*See also* Death penalty)
  juvenile delinquents, sentencing to life without parole, 79–80, 90, 93–94
  sex offenders, sentencing under different statute precluded without hearing, 163–164
Seventh Amendment, 197
Severe but rare inherent risks of medical procedures, liability for nondisclosure, 11

Sex Offender Registration and Notification Act of 2006, 163
Sex offenders, 163–168
  civil commitment beyond scheduled release date, 168, 184, 191
  double jeopardy, sexually violent predator statutes not violating prohibition against, 164–166, 192
  due process, sexually violent predator statutes not denial of, 165–166, 192
  ex post facto laws, sexually violent predator statutes not violating prohibition against, 164–166, 192
  incentives to participate in sexual abuse treatment program not violating self-incrimination privilege, 166–167, 185, 194
  proof of inability to control behavior not required, 167
  self-incrimination privilege and, 164, 166–167, 185
  sentencing under different statute precluded without hearing, 163–164
  sexually violent predator statute not criminal in nature, 164–165
Sexual harassment, 112–114
  definition of hostile work environment sexual harassment, 125, 127
  injury to psychological well-being not required for hostile environment sexual harassment, 113
  quid pro quo linkage not required, 112–113
  same-sex harassment, 114
  sexual desire, role of, 122
  unwelcomeness of advances, 123
Sexually violent predator statutes
  civil commitment procedure not violating constitutional protections, 165–166, 192
  not criminal in nature, 164–165, 182–183, 188
Sex with patients
  emotional harm caused by, 127
  as malpractice, 115
  malpractice insurance coverage, 105–106, 122
  physicians and, 105–106, 122
  psychotherapists and, 115, 122

Sixth Amendment
  admissibility of evidence from pretrial psychiatric evaluations, death penalty proceedings, 157
  competency to stand trial, effect of amnesia on, 136
  expert testimony under, 22
  informing suspects of rights, 131
  right to counsel, pretrial psychiatric evaluations, death penalty proceedings, 185
  self-representation, standard for, 140
  text of, 197
Sovereign immunity, ADA and, 102
Specific threat, duty to protect in absence of, 17–18
Spina bifida, catheterization during school hours for students with, 82–83
State, personal information collected by, 5
Subpoenas
  billing fraud, subpoena of records for, 7
  contempt for refusal to respond to, 5–6
Substituted judgment standard, guardians and right to refuse treatment, 55, 64, 68–69
Suicide, physician-assisted
  generally, 65–67
  due process right to, 49
  equal protection right to, 49–50
Supreme Court, path to, 201

Telecommunications, ADA and, 124
Tenth Amendment
  civil commitment and, 67
  text of, 197
Termination of parental rights, preponderance of evidence standard, 77, 89–93
Texas
  Department of Corrections, 151
  Department of Criminal Justice, 162
  Health Care Liability Act, 110
Third Amendment, 196
Third parties
  dangerous persons, duty to protect third parties from, 15–16, 33, 36, 38–39
  foreseeable but unidentified third parties, duty to protect, 16–17
  patient noncompliance with medication, duty to protect third parties from consequences of, 17
Title VII (Civil Rights Act of 1964)
  generally, 119
  definition of hostile work environment sexual harassment, 125, 127
  injury to psychological well-being not required for hostile environment sexual harassment, 113
  quid pro quo linkage not required for sexual harassment, 112–113
  same-sex sexual harassment under, 114
Tort law, 95–127
  generally, 95
  disabled persons, 97–102 (*See also* Disabled persons)
  emotional harm, 103–104 (*See also* Emotional harm)
  health insurance, 105–111 (*See also* Health insurance)
  malpractice (*See* Malpractice)
  questions, 116–127
  sex between psychotherapist and patient as malpractice, 115
  sexual harassment, 112–114 (*See also* Sexual harassment)
Treatment, right to. *See* Right to treatment
Trial, competency to stand. *See* Competency to stand trial

Ulster County (NY) Department of Social Services, 77
United States Courts of Appeals, geographic boundaries of, 204
United States Marshal Service, 6
United States Supreme Court, path to, 201
Utilization review
  ERISA preemption of state malpractice claims, 108, 110–111
  liability of health insurance for decisions in, 107–108

Vermont Act 114, 101, 117, 122–123
Veterans Administration, 16, 18
Victim impact statements, admissibility during sentencing in death penalty proceedings, 159, 191
Volitional element of insanity defense, 149–150, 190

Voluntary commitment, incompetent persons unable to consent to, 14, 36

Voluntary intoxication
due process, exclusion of evidence of voluntary intoxication and, 143, 185–186
murder charge, effect on, 142–143

Waiver
constitutional rights, standard for, 138–139
psychotherapist-patient privilege, 3–4

Washington Community Protection Act of 1990, 165

Weinstein, Henry, xxii

Wisconsin Department of Social Services, 75

Workers' compensation, compensability for emotional injuries under, 97–98, 124–125

Wright, J. Skelly, 54–55

Zone of danger for emotional harm, 123

www.ingramcontent.com/pod-product-compliance
Ingram Content Group UK Ltd.
Pitfield, Milton Keynes, MK11 3LW, UK
UKHW021329180426
11947UKWH00017B/1524